Did My Narcissistic Mother Love Me?

*Dealing with Manipulation &
Trauma from Narcissist –
Healing & Recovery of
Narcissism Abuse in Toxic, Abusive
Family Relationship with
Parents, Father or Mother*

Nanette Abigail

considered an endorsement from the trademark holder.

Table of Contents

Your Free Resource Is Awaiting

To better help you, I've created a simple mind map you can use *right away* to easily understand, quickly recall and readily use what you'll be learning in this book.

Click Here To Get Your Free Resource

Alternatively, here's the link:

https://viebooks.club/freeresourcemindmapfordidmynarcissisticmotherloveme

Your Free Resource Is Waiting..

Get Your Free Resource Now!

Introduction

Thank you for purchasing this book.

This book contains information, tips, and advice on recovery from narcissistic abuse. It is designed to be used by daughters of narcissistic mothers who may be looking for information on recovery and healing.

This book covers information on narcissism, its types, and its effects on daughters of mothers with NPD, or Narcissistic Personality Disorder. It offers information on possible root causes and effects of abuse, suggestions on how to handle them, the needs and challenges that one may face, and how such a woman can find newness of life in an ever-confusing world.

Much of the information and advice provided in this book is gleaned from my own personal experience. Recovery from narcissistic abuse, in my experience, was a roller coaster of a journey.

It was difficult for me to get out of a controlling relationship. I have to admit that I didn't have the strength or even the courage to get out of that relationship. The difficulty lay in the fact that the narcissist in my life was my mother.

In my young mind, I thought that you can't walk away from your mom—she's Mom, for goodness sake! And that, I think, is the unique situation with daughters of narcissistic mothers.

I went through the usual motions that occur to many daughters who have narcissistic moms.

I developed this affinity towards my mother. That was a totally polar reaction to that of my brother. He grew to hate Mom while I clung to the hope that maybe if I could be a little better, a bit prettier, or become politer, she would somehow come to give me the kind of love that I saw with other girls.

She would love me one moment and then hate me the next. It was so confusing. I thought I was going to lose my mind at certain points.

It took a long while before I had my very own "wake up call," and I talk about that in this book. Even then, after I had recognized that something was wrong and I was able to recognize that Mom was a narcissist, I still hoped that I could change her.

Long story short—I failed.

I had to learn how to set boundaries and create safe havens and ways to find mental clarity. I will be forever grateful for friends and family who loved me enough to rescue me from such an abusive relationship.

I am also thankful to the therapists who were patient with me. I derive a lot of insight from what I have learned through the therapy sessions I had and am still having with them.

We all need to take our first steps to healing and then overcome the aftereffects of such a crazy relationship. In this book, I also talk about how to deal with the anger, anxiety, and grief. I have included a few tools that were helpful to me, and I hope that they will be helpful to you, too.

Thanks for purchasing this book, I hope you enjoy it!

Chapter 1: Why is Recovering from a Narcissistic Relationship so Difficult?

Why is it so hard to recover from narcissistic abuse?

That is a huge question that gets asked a lot by people who had to exit relationships with someone who has a narcissistic personality. If you're the one going through this, then a lot of times, you will think long and hard about what was wrong with you.

In my case, there were plenty of times when I became desperate. I searched and grappled for approval. The thing is that you never notice that maybe it wasn't you who was to be blamed for all your suffering.

The things that you felt and the things that you experienced have a way to get back at you. They cling to you, and there are days when it seems that the good and the bad about your previous relationship tend to intertwine and your memory gets so mixed up that you can't tell which is which anymore.

Part of you is already telling you that you should be relieved that you just escaped from a relationship with your narcissistic mother, but a part of you will make you doubt that decision.

You would first think about all the good stuff that your mom has done, how she seemed to care and then you just couldn't believe how things got turned around—you can't even tell when everything went flipside.

Then there is that part of you that still wants to try to make amends with that narcissistic person you just escaped.

The Level of Intimacy is a Trap in Itself

Now, this is an interesting thing to wrap your mind around—do you remember how intimate your relationship was before your breakup? The more intimate the relationship was—say husband and wife or mother and daughter—the more difficult it was to get away from it.

That is the same thing with your relationship with a narcissistic mother—especially for daughters raised by a narcissistic mom. I had the most difficult time letting go in my mind because I felt that I had that special mother-daughter bond.

That is also true in other relationships. Even after many months later in a divorce, the wife would still be wondering how she would be able to recover from her losses. Those losses aren't just physical or financial. It entails that lost connection that you thought was already meant for the long-term.

A common pattern that you should be aware of is that initiation into the relationship. If you were the daughter of a narcissistic mom, your initiation started many years ago while you were still very young.

You were taught to believe in certain things— you're too fat, you'll never be near the worth of your mother, you are there to be adored by other people so that they will also make your mom happy, and others.

The initiatory process is so effective and gets so deeply rooted that it will be a monumental struggle before you can even learn to cope with the abuse that has been conditioned into your mind.

Narcissists are Also Trapped in Their Own Paradox

Now, this might sound insane, but it's actually a piece of cold hard truth. It's a love-hate relationship that gets played over and over in your head.

Narcissists go through the same motions as well. It is definitely hard to believe, but that is the grand truth. They might hate you or at least act like they hate you but then they also miss you and want you back in their lives.

Do you notice how someone with a narcissistic tendency sort of finds their way back to you? They send you text messages, they leave you emails, and they might even just show up one fine day knocking at your door for no reason at all. They do that when you least expect it.

You have divorced your narcissistic husband, you now have your own family and left your narcissistic mother, and yet they will try in their own little way to get in touch with you. It'll drive you nuts.

Author of *Rethinking Narcissism*, Dr. Craig Malkin, says that people who have NPD (Narcissistic Personality Disorder) are sort of trapped themselves. He says that narcissists are caught up in a "constant battle between wanting you and pushing you away."

The big difference between you and the narcissist you were in a relationship with is in the manner of manifesting such inner conflict. For most of us who have been there, we tend to go through a fit of anxiety and at times cry about it for a while.

A narcissist will express or manifest it in the most insane way ever. They will send you an email, for instance. At first you will think that they want to reconnect. They might even write kind words in that email. However, you will also get disparaging remarks when you actually go through the entire text.

Remember that a relationship is a two-way street. When it is no longer that way, you exit the relationship. The narcissist might want that, too. However, you want your exit to have meaningful closure. The narcissist, on the other hand, won't go down without a fight. Needless to say, you both want the same thing, but you just have a different idea or concept on how you want the relationship to end.

Four Impact Points That Make Recovery So Hard

The following are four big reasons why recovery from a narcissistic relationship is so difficult:

1. *The loving relationship you remembered wasn't real*

This is kind of devastating, especially for a child. Someone once wisely said that a daughter who was raised by a narcissistic mother never really experienced the love of a mother after all. In fact, some even go so far as to say that such children never really had a mother at all.

There was no mother-daughter relationship to begin with. They weren't two dancing the proverbial tango. It was just the narcissistic mom doing all the dancing in the spotlight by herself. There was no "me and Mom" thing—you never had a "thing" with your mom; it was just her. You were just a tool that she could use so she could bask in the limelight.

Once you come to terms with this truth, then recovery can begin. You can revisit each moment that you had with your mother—all the good things you thought were there You will then start to realize why she did or said those things to you. It was all to bring things back to her.

2. *She made you doubt yourself*

If you looked really hard, you should have noticed all the red flags in your relationship. In hindsight, you would think that you should have seen them right from the start, but you didn't.

One expert explains that there is a dizzying thing that narcissists do to people around them—they play mind games with them. You missed all the signals simply because you were trapped in a tangle of lies and deceit.

You were told a web of half-truths so much that you began to doubt yourself. You have doubted your memory and questioned your own judgment. You had that gut feeling that something was wrong, but you ended up thinking that it was you that was wrong. Some have even succumbed to paranoia.

It takes a lot of effort to uncover one lie only to discover another one. You will have to take every effort to try and connect the dots. All the while, you will realize this crushing fact—you colluded with your narcissistic mother. You were an accomplice in her schemes.

Somehow, in your innocence and self-doubt, you helped her win. That is a lot to take in. Realizing that might make you relive every emotional moment over and over as it eats you up inside.

3. *You feel like a fool*

Insecurity brews up inside us as we uncover the lies we lived with and we begin to doubt ourselves. Getting over it all isn't easy because the moment you free yourself from all the mental manipulation, you drag yourself into one—this one you made yourself:

You feel like you've made a fool of yourself.

That's just as bad as being manipulated with lies and mental games. A lot of people fall into self-criticism. They begin to ascribe the bad things that happened in their lives to the deficiencies they have observed in their character.

What they should have seen is a series of missteps that ordinary people make. Well, it's kind of complicated when those mistakes were compounded by the influence of a narcissist pulling on the proverbial reins.

It takes time and effort to realize that you were played simply because you were naïve and innocent. You were an inexperienced soul under the manipulations of a master mentalist. What chance could you have ever had against such odds?

Experts confirm that self-blame is a common phenomenon in people who have been through a narcissistic relationship. You have somehow convinced yourself that all you ever needed to do was to be a better daughter and maybe, just maybe, Mother would approve and love you because you were able to change. That line of thinking eventually erodes a person's self-esteem.

4. *Feeling powerless*

After taking all the abuse from a narcissistic mother, one would start to feel powerless. You see, a narcissist will do everything to maintain control, and if she has control, what do you have? You are left with no options—you feel powerless to make any changes to your circumstances.

There is no chance at proactivity here when that happens. You also have very little chance at attaining an emotional balance simply because someone else controls the ins and outs of a relationship and you have no say in it.

Some people carry this feeling of powerlessness all the way to adulthood. They live in fear and anxiety, struggling to please people but not getting any desired results from the effort.

The hard and fast truth here is that you can get over a narcissistic relationship with your mother.

You're a survivor.

Don't forget that. You are a strong woman. You escaped the biggest monster of your life and that means something. It also means you can heal. You can thrive. You can live a happy, productive, and satisfying life as an independent person.

And the good news is that the power was in you all along.

That's what we are going to cover in the next chapter.

Chapter 2: That Intriguing Wakeup Call—Your Psychological Immune System

Just like your body has an immune system to fight off the toxic, infectious, and damaging bacteria, viruses, and germs, the mind also has something akin to it. Daniel Gilbert, a psychologist from the Psychology Department of Harvard University, called it the Psychological Immune System.

So, what is it? It is that part of your mind that kicks in after being exposed to psychological trauma. For a lot of people, this vital part of the mind kicks in after the conflict has washed over— that is, after all the tears have been cried and all the shouting matches have concluded.

You can say that this is that part of you that tells you all the things that have gone wrong in that relationship that you initially thought was all well and good. This thing works like a natural signaling system.

Gilbert says that it kicks in after a moment of calm. It's that short moment when you're done crying and loathing yourself. You then experience a feeling of detachment that you no longer have that bond with your narcissistic mother.

Give It a Boost

That's when all the bad things start to add up. That is when you finally make sense of things and have the will to start over with your life. However, before you can begin to start over, your psychological immune system will need a boost.

Why do you need to give your mind's immune system a boost?

Well, recovering from a narcissistic relationship will be so much more difficult compared to recovering from a normal broken relationship with a spouse, parent, or some other loved one. Why is that?

For starters, there was no love to begin with.

Recovering from a relationship with a husband who left you for another woman is easier to get away from. At least you have something to remember him by. You can say to yourself that there was something in your relationship and he at least loved you for a time.

Getting over the loss of a parent is easy for just the same reason. Your mom may have left you and your dad for another guy, but you know you still have that connection to her. You can still call her mom and no matter what, she will still love you because you are her child.

It's like you have a base or a foundation to work with, which helps your psychological immune system get by.

But you don't have that when you're trying to get over a relationship with a narcissistic mother.

There was no love to begin with. That makes it all a lot harder.

Some have compared the recovery process to recovering from war shock. In fact, while you're in the process of recovering from one, you might still be fighting and struggling against the continuous tactics used by a person with Narcissistic Personality Disorder.

Recovering from narcissistic "love" is more like recovering from an actual disease—a really bad sickness, something rather life-threatening. But this time, it's not a virus, bacteria, or anything that's trying to infect and destroy you.

What are trying to get to you from the inside are hurt feelings, resentment, and anger. They're the things that try to eat you up inside. With betrayal and hurt going down this deep, sometimes you find it hard to trust yourself. It needs a regular conscious choice to rise above.

The good news is that there are several things that you can do to help your psychological immune system. We will only touch a little on these techniques here; we'll cover them and other coping mechanisms in more detail in later chapters.

Here are the four things that you can do to give your psychological immune system a boost:

1. Use Cool Processing

Cool and hot processing or cool and hot cognitions are distinctions made in different types of psychological research. It is studied in such fields as neuropsychology, social psychology, clinical psychology, cognitive psychology, and a lot of others.

Let's go over these two concepts a little deeper. The idea behind this hypothesis is that human beings process their decisions as they are influenced (or the lack thereof) by their emotional states.

Hot processing is when we process our ideas and make our decisions as we are influenced by our current emotional state. When we are cold processing, our decisions and responses to what others say or do (or have said or have done) is not affected or influenced by our emotions. You need to practice cool processing.

Here's a simple way you can do that. Whenever you recall a feeling that you had with your narcissistic mom, maybe how you feel when you recall a particular experience with her, think about the why rather than the what. For example, you remembered that feeling of helplessness from the way your mom reacted when you arrived home from grade school crying really hard because a classmate bullied you. She gets angry with you instead of giving you comfort and hugs. With this childhood experience, try to think about why you feel that way.

What I mean to say is that it is really easy to focus on what you were feeling during such an experience as stated above. It takes effort and some distancing—a reverse of empathizing, instead of putting yourself in those shoes, you move out of them. You step back and try to observe yourself in that situation.

You already know what you were feeling. Now it's time to focus on why you were feeling that emotion. Research shows that your emotional intelligence is improved the more you understand your emotions. Eventually you will learn how to identify each emotion more precisely, and that gives you some form of leverage when you're trying to manage your emotions.

One way to do this is to try and imagine those events happening to someone else. Imagine that someone else is feeling the same emotions you have felt after going through the same experience as you did. Now, try to recall why you felt that way. Why you felt helpless, why you felt like you were useless, why you felt powerless. When you understand the why, you will be able to work out how to get over the source of the emotion rather than be influenced by said emotion.

2. Personalize the Experience and Do Not Generalize

One common phenomenon for people who have been through narcissistic abuse is to generalize everything. They go from my mom is a mean person to all mothers are mean.

Here's one thing you can do to avoid falling into that trap. Always personalize all the issues that you are going through. When your mother made her evening poker games more important than you—thus leaving you home every night—she was the only mother who did that to you.

The other mothers didn't have a clue what was happening. When your mother ridiculed you by telling you how ugly or fat you looked, it was only her who said that. The other mothers in the room didn't say that. There was only one bad apple in the entire orchard—the rest of the apples were fine.

3. Compassion for the Self

Another thing that you can do to help give your psychological immune system a boost is to practice self-compassion. For someone who has been through constant traumatizing experiences with a narcissistic mother, going down into an ocean of self-criticism is such an easy thing. You can turn things around using a three-step process:

a. *Start by being kind to yourself.* You're not stupid and you're not worthless. Sure, you made mistakes, and who hasn't? Think along these lines: the first person to be kind to you is yourself, and you can't expect anyone to be kind to you—not even your narcissistic mom, so do yourself a favor and be kind and forgiving. Your mistakes are stepping stones to better times ahead.

b. *Second, see things with an eternal perspective.* We're not referring to anything spiritual by that. What I was actually trying to emphasize is to take a really long-term perspective of your life.

Realize that your initial experience living with a narcissistic mother is only a small portion of your life if you consider the eternal scheme of things. Notice that you're not the first person nor are you the last person to ever make mistakes.

There is a lifetime waiting to happen and it's exciting. The lessons you learned from your experience with your narcissistic mother is the universe telling you to move forward and upward. Your suffering and the mistakes you made are too small in comparison to the good that you will eventually do. That good will not only affect your life but the lives of others long after you are gone.

c. *You are not your pain. You are not your feelings.* Sometimes we lose sight of the reality in this life that your feelings and all the pain you feel are not you. They're a tiny fraction of your human experience.

Of course, you should be aware of your feelings. However, you should never iden-

tify with them to the point that your feelings own you and not the other way
around. Later in this book, we'll go over
something called mindfulness to help you
draw that line between you and your emotions.

4. Always Take the High Road

Your narcissistic mother just can't get enough of
you. Even if you have separated yourself from her,
you already have a husband and kids, your mom
will still find ways to inject herself into your life's
equation. That's how hard it is to stay away from
a narcissistic mom.

That is why you should make it a practice to always take the high road. Expect to get the same
old treatment. Expect to be badmouthed. Expect
to be humiliated in front of other people. Expect
a lot of bad things to happen next time you meet—
she will still be insufferable, and it would be asking too much to hope that she would have
changed a bit.

Make a record of your new interactions. Lashing
back against her, especially in public, will sort of

feel good. Well, for a little while, anyway. But then it's easy to fall into that trap and your narcissistic mom will have you backtracking and defending yourself all over again.

Why shouldn't you engage your narcissistic mom in a war of words? Well, for one thing, that is exactly what she wants. If you do not react, then she couldn't pull any strings like the proverbial puppeteer that she is.

Part of the high road is to forgive her. Forgiveness might take a bit to come along. It will come, but it will require a huge amount of emotional intellect and maturity on your part. It's the child who must practice some "adulting" instead of the parent.

But doing so will do you all the benefits. It may not help your narcissistic mother, but it will help you to recover—and that is what really matters at the end of the day.

In the next chapter, we'll go over what narcissism is, Narcissistic Personality Disorder, and what goes on in the mind of the narcissist. Understanding how a narcissist thinks will help you understand why your mother did what she did to you.

It may also help you eventually get over her antics and maybe find closure.

Chapter 3: The Narcissistic Mindset

We will not mention the actual names of the women whose stories we will tell below. In fact, their own testimonies have been edited so as not to mention real people's names, places, events, etc. They were more than helpful to share a part of their life stories, and we wouldn't want to poke into their actual private lives. It is my hope that you will get insights into the narcissistic mindset in the stories of these women—girls who grew up with a narcissistic mother.

Here is Vicky's story:

"I grew up thinking I wasn't really good enough—for anything. I couldn't even dare to consider doing ballet when I was a young girl even though a lot of the kids in the neighborhood were already taking ballet lessons.

Mother always told me I was such a klutz that I would make a fool of myself. The infuriating part was that I believed that I was like that.

My art teacher once time told me I was good at drawing. I couldn't believe her because mother told me otherwise.

One day, I found something I was good at—swimming. I tried and my dad supported me somewhat, but he wasn't always there. He was always busy with work.

With Dad's blessing, I took swimming lessons. My mom, on the other hand, did more than frown on my decision. I found something that I was good at and my swim coach even said that she wanted to help train me for some competition.

I never showed up for practice. Eventually I quit swimming altogether. My mother convinced me that I will just end up embarrassing myself come competition day. The sad thing was that I believed her.

I hoped that letting her know that I found something that I was really good at would make her proud of me. Instead, she told me off and made me quit.

In fact, she made me quit every time I tried something new."

Key Takeaways: To a narcissistic mother, you are never good enough. You can try to please her. You can try your best to please her but nothing you do works. However, she will instead make you do the things that she wants you to do and stay under her shadow, figuratively speaking.

To a narcissistic mother, control over you is everything. That boosts her self-esteem. When you do something of your own accord and against her wishes she will do what she can to make you change your mind and eventually doubt yourself.

Why? Because when you start to embrace independence, she loses control. Control is everything to her.

Here is Angela's story:

"The world was such a confusing place when I was a little girl. I think it is still quite confusing now that I am an adult. At home I was told by my mother, and to a certain degree by my dad, that I was deeply flawed and I needed their guidance.

However, when I'm at school, my teachers always tell me how great a student I was. I always told them that I was that good because of my mom. They thought that it was so cute and that I was such a humble girl.

They didn't understand that I wasn't being either. I was actually just parroting exactly what my mother wanted me to say.

Then a paradox happened. My teacher one day gave us a math problem. I can't remember the details, but it had something to do with measuring the height of a table when all we knew was the height of a glass of water and the height of a chair—something like that.

We had the hardest time solving it but then I had that sudden stroke of genius—I had an idea. I didn't know where it came from. My mom never taught me any math, for goodness sake.

I remember walking to the board and writing down my solution.

It was brilliant! Well, my teacher said so. My classmates cheered me on. For the first time in my life, I felt how it was like to be appreciated by people.

I remember coming home that day telling Mother all about it.

She said, "Oh, you fooled the lot of them, didn't you!" She even laughed hysterically as if it was the funniest thing in the world.

It was one of the happiest and saddest days of my young life."

Key Takeaways: A narcissistic mother will want you to believe that you can't do anything without her. She wants you to depend on her and, to an extreme, beg for her approval—something that will never come.

What you experience outside of the home will always be different from what happens inside the home. She will use different mind games on you. She will lie, she will cover things up, she will make fun of you, and she will turn your best effort into a joke. She will never want you to have the upper hand.

Here is Ayesha's Story:

"It was a hard lesson for me when I was a little girl. I learned early that I didn't have to worry about my little brothers from

coming into my room and rummaging through my stuff.

Well, they did that a lot, but it was just harmless musings. They were more interested in jumping on my bed and playing tag or playing those pro wrestling games they love to play.

Oh yeah, they always make a mess of my room every time they find a way to open the door. It was either I end up cleaning my room or I would be yelling and screaming at them and then they leave in a flash and I end up cleaning my room anyway.

But my two little brothers were the least of my worries.

I found out the hard way that it was my mother who I had to worry about. One day, I asked those two how they got in and they frankly told me Mother went in, so they thought it was okay.

Later on, I found out that Mother went through most of my personal stuff and paid special attention to my diary. She read through every page.

On top of that, she was upset. She was angry that I was 'keeping secrets' from her. That wasn't the worst thing about it. I also learned that her going into my room was a regular thing."

Key Takeaways: Don't expect a narcissistic mother to respect your personal boundaries. There is no such thing as my room, my closet, my diary, my stuff with her. She does not respect such boundaries because to her there is none. In her eyes, she has all the right to bulldozer her way into your life.

She has no respect for boundaries because she cannot distinguish the unique individuals in her children. In her eyes, they are but extensions or even reflections of herself. This trait is an inevitable compromise in her ability for parenthood.

The Following is Tiffany's Story

"I really thought that breaking up with my boyfriend was the hardest thing in the world. [He] was a nice guy—or so I thought. He was so sweet all the time that I never noticed that he was cheating on me.

Of course, when I found out, I was devastated. I really thought he loved me.

I didn't let my mom know because I knew that she would be upset—to say the least. I was smiling around other people, especially at home. I didn't let my sisters know and I didn't let my parents know.

I looked and acted like the coolest person in the world, just like what Mom wanted me to be. But deep down inside and behind every smile were a lot of bottled up emotions.

A few days later, I couldn't keep it in anymore, so I told my best friend [name withheld].

Later that day, I went home, and Mom was upset. She then cried and told me that she felt betrayed and that I had betrayed her. She said that my best friend called and told her everything.

I never blamed her for telling Mom since she never knew what my mother was capable of. Then I let it all out and confessed to Mother. "Oh, so now you tell me?" Then she goes on about how I hurt her and how I victimized her. She totally ignored the fact that I was hurting from my breakup. She then went into a breakdown, which made my dad angry when he got home.

The fact that I was emotionally hurting got brushed aside and everything was my fault."

Key Takeaways: A narcissistic mother has no ability to empathize with her daughter. When you reach out calling to her for your needs, those requests will be dismissed as non-consequential and unimportant.

To show you just how insignificant your cries for help are, she will be a towering authority dismissing everything you say as irrelevant. She can also do the exact opposite, she will play as the victim, ignoring the fact that you desperately needed something from her. The attention passes from you to her and she has to be the center of everything.

Sometimes a narcissistic mother may also have married a narcissistic father.

This One is from Amy:

"My mom always bought me the prettiest dresses. You can say that she made me look like a cute little doll. She did that a lot and on many occasions.

She dolled me up not only during holidays or special occasions like my birthday or something. She did it even if she just wanted to take a walk in the park. She usually would comment that I should look nice just in case we bump into one of her friends.

Guess what? We seemed to always run into a few of her friends. It happened every single time. So, how did I fit in with the grown-ups?

They would adore how good I look. They would usually say the nicest things about me. Every time that happened, she would grab all the glory. I was pretty because of her. I was such a polite girl because of her. She was the reason for all that was good about me."

Key Takeaways: A narcissistic mother loves to doll up her daughter, and she does it for the wrong reasons. She teaches her daughter to be polite, not because it is the right thing to do but because it will make her look good in eyes of the public. Anything good achieved by the daughter is a reflection of the narcissistic mother.

This is Nora's Story

"My mother always told me that I was headstrong and I defied her every wish. I really never identified with my mother. I

always felt that there was a power struggle between us.

My father loved me and treated me kindly. But now that I think about it after decades of hindsight, it was like whenever my dad did something nice for me, my mother would get angry and jealous.

The day I left for college was a big sigh of relief for me. My mother always wanted me to study at the nearby college. But I chose to study out of state. She then said the most outrageous things like I had it good here. They would have paid for my rent but now I will have to pay rent on top of tuition and other fees. She said, 'You will one day see how good you could have had it here' or something to that effect.

Well, as it turned out, I could really do it all on my own. Yes, I'm still paying for my student loan. But it's still something to celebrate—I graduated on my own blood, sweat, and tears. My dad was really happy for me and was there for me all the time.

But Mother never showed up for my grad-uation.

I landed my first job and that made my daddy proud. My mom, on the other hand, side commented complaining about why young kids get the better jobs nowa-days. She even claims that the only reason I landed such a good job was because she raised me with high self-esteem. She even pointed out that I should be thankful for her."

Key Takeaways: Narcissistic mothers jealously fight for attention. She gets offended when you go against her wishes. She gets jealous of your achievements.

Common Experiences of Daughters Raised by Narcissistic Mothers

In this section, we'll cover all the most common experiences of daughters who were raised by narcissistic mothers. Later on, we will cover the symptoms of Narcissistic Personality Disorder (NPD).

Note that the symptoms of this condition will vary in their severity. Nevertheless, there are common threads in the experiences of those daughters who have lived with a mother with NPD.

1. Lack of boundaries

Note that the effects of a narcissistic mother on a daughter are a lot different from a son. Why? Well, for one thing, daughters tend to spend more time with their mothers than sons. Daughters tend to look up to their moms and see them as the role model.

The lack of boundaries between mother and daughter ruins a huge part of that relationship. Narcissistic mothers see their daughters as nothing more than annexes to their very own egos. On the flipside, which is kind of crazy, they also see their daughters as threats.

Living with them is like a double-edged sword. You switch from their good sides to their bad sides and back with just a snap of their fingers. The mood swings are sometimes so unbearable.

They use criticism as well as instruction or direction to change their daughter. The end goal, of course, is to create their daughter into a version of themselves. Well, to be exact, the ideal version of themselves—the version they couldn't achieve themselves.

The crazy thing about this is that while they shape their daughters into who they would have wanted themselves to be, they also project their own unwanted aspects on their child. That is why they use coldness, obstinacy, and self-centeredness.

2. Competition

Believe it or not, sometimes living with a narcissistic mother is a lot like Snow White. Your mother is the evil queen who believes and often tells herself that she is the fairest of them all.

The sad part is that the lovely daughter is always in some sort of competition with her mother. In the mother's eyes, she is competing with her daughter for Daddy's love. If not, then it's the son's love or someone else's.

She might appear protective of her daughter. She would even go as far as to disparage her daughter's boyfriend. She might even restrict them from seeing one another. She might even say that the guy isn't good enough for her daughter.

Motive is everything if you want to decipher the narcissistic mother's actions. Sure, she might want to protect her daughter—that's what she wants you to see. But what she really wants is totally something else.

She invades her daughter's privacy. She might even undermine any other relationships that she is having like friends, neighbors, best friends, and even flirt with the guys that her daughter knows.

3. Control

You can say that a narcissistic mother is myopic in that they see that the world revolves around them. They control and manipulate not only their children's choices. They also manipulate their feelings as well as their needs.

They will even take it against them when they can't exercise this control over them. They even

think that the kids deserve some form of punish-
ment when that happens. Sometimes the control
that a narcissistic mother exerts is absolute and,
in her best management, she focuses on her son
and neglects her daughter.

There are narcissistic mothers who will insist that
their daughters should always look their best and
behave the best way they can. However, the defi-
nition of what is best is always up to the mother
and not the daughter.

She might tell you that she is doing it only for your
own good. They expect compliance as well as
gratitude. However, all this attention also leads to
the mother's envy of the good things that the
daughter has received or achieved.

4. They are emotionally unavailable

There is no such thing as maternal tenderness for
a narcissistic mother. Sure, they might be able to
provide for their daughter's physical needs, but
she will be emotionally unavailable.

This would leave the child confused, and she will
never be able to realize what she was missing. She

sees the loving and warmth that her friends and other relatives experience from their mothers, but she never experiences any of that. She longs for understanding and she longs for warmth but never gets it.

Thus, that mother-daughter connection is never created. She yearns for that connection, but it is either just a fleeting experience or is something that is totally absent. It's something that is absolutely elusive to her.

So, what is left to the daughter? She is left with emptiness—a void that never gets filled and it grows inside of her. She then senses an anxiety growing inside of her, an anxiety for something that has always been missing in her life. She will attempt to fill that void inside of her through relationships with friends, coworkers, and others. Yet that emotional emptiness remains, and it sometimes gets repeated over and over.

5. Toxic shaming

A daughter who is raised by a narcissistic mother rarely or never feels accepted. She is also unaccepted for being who she really is, which means she can't be herself. She is always forced to make a choice between losing her mommy's love and sacrificing herself.

When she displays who her true self is, she is often shamed. All of that is a ploy forcing her into a state of self-denial. First her true self is denied by her narcissistic mother, and then she finally denies it herself.

Later in life, this toxic shaming can get compounded by feelings of hatred and anger. This daughter will direct that anger first on her mother, yet she accepts the fact that maybe all the criticisms that her mother made might be true.

She strives to do her best, yet she lacks that feeling of fulfillment. In her relationships as an adult, she might repeat the cycle of abandonment all over again. She tends to leave before the other fellow leaves her—it's inevitable anyway. It now becomes her defensive fence against pain, resentment, and further possible shaming.

Outcome

As we can see from the experiences shared by the women above and the descriptions provided after, narcissistic abuse includes a huge amount of control and repeated shaming. They undermine the young girl's identity and later on create low self-esteem and insecurity.

The young girl starts to believe that it is her fault—for everything, including why her mother is displeased with her. She no longer trusts her own feelings or her female impulses.

Some daughters come to believe that they should never have been born. Some feel that they are a burden to their mothers. The fathers of daughters raised by narcissistic mothers are seldom of any help at all. They could be passive or more of an absentee parent than anything.

Chapter 4: Narcissism, NPD, and Narcissus

Who is Narcissus?

To further help with the understanding of narcissism, we will touch slightly on the origin of this term. Narcissism comes from Greek mythology, specifically from the tale of Narcissus.

Narcissus was a hunter by profession, which is according to John Tzetzes, a Byzanitine poet, who lived in the 12th century. Some sources say that he was from Thespiae in Boeotia. He is the type of guy who despised those who loved him, yet he loved all things that are beautiful.

The myth of Narcissus actually has several versions, but the story goes this way. One day, Narcissus was walking in the woods and then a nymph called Echo saw him. She immediately fell deeply in love with him and she followed him around.

Narcissus, being the great hunter that he was, noticed that there was someone following him. He then shouted, "Who's there?" Echo did not reveal herself but only echoed his words, saying "who's there."

However, she couldn't hold herself back and finally revealed herself. She immediately tried to embrace him, but he stepped back. He also told the nymph to leave him alone, which broke her heart.

She lived the rest of her life alone and lonely. She remained in that state until there was nothing left of her but echoing sounds. The goddess of revenge known as Nemesis decided to exact vengeance on Narcissus.

One summer day, Narcissus got thirsty after hunting all day. The goddess lured him into the water. In the water, he saw his own reflection and fell in love with it deeply.

He couldn't remove his gaze from his reflection, well, all versions of this myth agree on this part. The rest of the story or the consequence of his actions is where the versions go in different places.

Some versions tell us that Narcissus got so absorbed by the beauty of his image that he kept staring into the water until nothing was left of him but the water plant called the daffodil or, in the Greek language, the narcissus plant.

Some versions have it that Narcissus got so frustrated about the fact that he couldn't consummate the love that he had that he committed suicide.

The key details of the story include the fact that Narcissus fell in love with himself, ergo the self-adoration and the self-fixation that we see among narcissists as well as the fact that he couldn't reciprocate the same love to Echo.

What happened to Echo? Due to her heartbroken state, she eventually became what we call the echo because of her capability to repeat other people's words over and over again. It's almost poetic how the daughter of a narcissistic mother can become her mother's echo as well, groomed to be another her that is only meant to be seen and never heard, let alone outshine her mother, should she not escape her situation in time.

Narcissism as It Is Used in Psychology

The words narcissism and narcissist are used in the world of psychology to describe someone who has a pathological fixation with oneself either in public perception or in one's appearance.

Back in 1898, sexologist Havelock Ellis used the term to refer to people who are habitual masturbators. Paul Nache in 1899 classified the habit as a sexual perversion and called it narcissism.

A psychoanalytical paper published in 1911 was published by Otto Rank [1]. This paper was focused on self-admiration and vanity, which were also termed as narcissism. In 1914, Sigmund Freud published his paper entitled "On Narcissism: An Introduction" [2].

The personality disorder related to this is called NPD or Narcissistic Personality Disorder. This disorder is one that is long-term and involves an excessive need for admiration, feelings of self-importance, and a distinct lack of empathy.

Overview and Symptoms

NPD or Narcissistic Personality Disorder is one of a few types of personality disorders classified in different branches of psychology. Someone who has this type of mental condition will have inflated sense of his personal worth even to the point of breaking with reality.

A person who has NPD also feels that he or she is really important and will have an excessive need for admiration or at least more attention from people. These people also characteristically lack any form of empathy for others.

All of that is a mask or what we may call a defense. What are these people trying to desperately hide and defend? A vulnerable self-esteem that is so fragile it breaks at the smallest kind of criticism.

The symptoms of NPD manifest themselves in social interactions. Often, the psychological condition causes a lot of trouble in the person's financial, school, work, and other relationships.

They will get disappointed when they are not given special favors at work, which they feel they actually deserve. The same is true if they do not get the admiration they expect from other people.

If the object of their attention is someone who they see is of a lower status than they are, then they will treat that other person as inferior and incidental to the benefits that they should obtain. They will manipulate them and control such people (usually their spouses, children, and other members of the family or anyone within their circle of influence).

It is also interesting that people with NPD can turn out to be good bosses. Well, they're already proficient at bossing people around. They're the ones who are really competitive and really hate losing. So, they push themselves and push other people at work and they will get results one way or another.

That is why they can actually make great managers. At the end of the day, the credit for all the success that has been gained by the company should be attributed to them—or so they think.

Symptoms of Narcissistic Personality Disorder

The following are the most common signs and symptoms of people with NPD. Note, however, that the severity of the manifestations of these symptoms will vary from one person to the next.

That means that you don't need to have all the symptoms listed below to be diagnosed with NPD. You can have as few as 3 to 5 symptoms and still be considered as having NPD.

Here are the symptoms:

- One who insists on and feels privileged into getting the best of everything.

- Usually behaves arrogantly. One with NPD will come across as someone who is pretentious, boastful, and conceited.

- A person with NPD will feel that others are envious of them but at the same time will be envious of others as well.

- Characteristically unwilling to recognize the needs of other people—including their children or spouses. They are unable to relate to the plight of other people affected by their actions.

- They tend to take advantage of people when they can and as long as they can get what they want.

- They expect you to give unquestioning compliance.

- They expect to receive special favors from others.

- They tend to monopolize every conversation that they get involved in.

- People with NPD also tend to look down on people who they believe are inferior to them. Expect them to belittle that person's work and value.

- These people often believe that they are so superior to others that they only associate with other people whom they perceive as equally superior as they are.

- They are often overpowered by their own fantasies of brilliance, beauty, power, and success even if they haven't proven themselves or achieved it yet for themselves.

- They are also preoccupied about fantasies of their perfect mate.

- They also tend to exaggerate when they relate their talents and achievements.

- These people also tend to expect some form of validation or recognition as being someone who is superior.

- They have a constant sense of entitlement.

- Their sense of self-importance is exaggerated.

Note that those aren't the only symptoms that will manifest in a person with NPD. Remember that they love to dish out criticisms but they also have trouble taking criticisms themselves. Sometimes what you say may not actually be a critique at all—

it could just be a passing comment or observation—and the person with NPD will immediately interpret it as a critique.

It is interesting to note of their reactions to such statements, which might include any of the following:

- They would have difficulty controlling their behavior or their feelings.

- Express or reveal secret feelings such as humiliation, vulnerability, shame, and insecurity.

- They will become moody.

- They will feel depressed due to the fact that they have fallen short of expectations or at extreme cases falling short of perfection.

- When pressed, a person with NPD might react with rage.

- They may also act superior and criticize back with full contempt. All of that is a ploy so that they will appear superior again compared to the person who they see is criticizing them.

- They also easily feel that they have been slighted even for the smallest thing.

- They will have interpersonal problems—a significant amount of that.

- A person with NPD will become angry and impatient when criticized or when the special treatment they were expecting wasn't provided to them.

Possible Complications

Narcissistic personality disorder does have serious possible complications when left untreated for prolonged periods of time. Again, several factors will contribute to the possible complications, and it doesn't mean that if you discover your mom to have the aforementioned narcissistic tendencies that she will develop the complications mentioned below.

Possible complications include the following:

- Suicidal behavior and thoughts

- Drug misuse

- Alcoholism

- Physical health problems

- Anxiety

- Depression

- Problems at school

- Problems in the workplace

- Relationship difficulties with a spouse that may eventually end in divorce or breakup.

Extreme Narcissism

It should be noted here that narcissism manifests itself in a continuum or grades of different expressions. On the one end, you have healthy self-esteem, and on the extreme end, you have an exaggerated sense of self-worth. That means some narcissists can be okay at some points and they can be rude, self-centered, and un-empathetic or unsympathetic at other points.

Extreme narcissists also differ from one another. Nevertheless, they still demonstrate their toxic personalities, always hedging up their grandiose self-image but in a variety of expressions. The following are what Dr. Joseph Burgo, Ph.D., a psychotherapist, calls the five extreme narcissists:

1. **The Grandiose Narcissist**: this is the more familiar kind of narcissist that you hear about. She always brags about her accomplishments and how great a person she is. We'll cover more details about this type of narcissist when we go over the standard classifications of people with Narcissistic Personality Disorder.

   So how do you deal with a grandiose narcissist? When this type of narcissist starts to assert her superiority, you will feel the urge to react, counter what she says, or even compete. Wrong move; that's exactly what she wants—don't fall for it. Just let her blow her steam and ignore her.

   Sometimes a grandiose narcissist will be very charismatic. She will draw in people who will want to emulate her or at least benefit from her superiority. Don't fall for that, either—she is trying to drag in admirers who don't really have that much value to her but only to boost her own ego.

2. **The Know-It-All**: this is the type of narcissist who is always highly opinionated and speaks her mind on the subject even if it is unsolicited. This is the kind of person who believes she knows it all. They always have a hard time listening to you because they're too preoccupied thinking about what they will say next.

   How to deal with a know-it-all type of narcissist? You have a choice between just ignoring the rant or dismissing the lecture (even if the narcissist is just halfway into his elaborate speech) with a polite and gentle "thank you for that information" and then move on to something else.

   You should be open (or at least try to appear that way) to her views but never endorse them. Never challenge their opinions or else you're in for a long lecture.

3. **The Seductive Narcissist**: this type of extreme narcissist will lure you in and even make you feel like you're a great person. She might even idolize you and make you feel like you're number one in all things.

It's a trap.

The goal of this extreme narcissist is to use you once you have been seduced. She will make you feel the same way about her, as if there is a common attraction or compelling bond between you two. Once she gets what she wants, then you get the cold shoulder and you get dumped.

How to deal with a seductive narcissist? Be humble and don't let flattery, admiration, and other means of seduction get to you. Observe the narcissist in her interactions with others and see her callous ways. That's how they really treat others— that's going to be you someday after the extreme narcissist is done with you.

4. **The Bully**: this type builds up her self-esteem by putting other people down and humiliating them. This type of extreme narcissist is more brutal than the first three types we have mentioned above. She uses contempt to make other people feel like losers. This kind of extreme narcissist has a really toxic personality. She belittles other people and mocks them.

How to deal with a bullying narcissist? Stay away from the bully and don't challenge her position unless you are absolutely sure that you can handle the physical violence. You might also have to report this one to the authorities if that is possible. The peaceful way out is to just avoid ruffling her overinflated ego. Stay out of her way and let her live in her own delusional world.

5. **The Vindicator**: this is the type of extreme narcissist that you should stay away from at all costs. Cross the line with this type of narcissist and she will devote many years of her life to finding a way to destroy

you. This is the type of narcissist that will try to destroy your reputation in the eyes of the public.

If you have a vindictive narcissist as your coworker and you challenge her ego, don't be surprised if she finds a way to get you fired. This one will trash-talk about you in front of your coworkers and even to your boss.

If your ex-wife is a vindictive narcissist, then don't be surprised to have a grueling custody battle. She can even spend many years trying to turn your own children against you. If she can, then she will try her best to get you tied up in the proceedings in family court.

How do you deal with a vindicator? Stay away from them. Cut ties if you have to. This type of extreme narcissist is the one you have to steer clear of at all costs. They damage other people's psyche as well as their reputation.

When you have one that is already hell-bent on you, then you should use legal actions—nothing less than a legalistic approach will work. Note that they can be very good at disguising who they are and their real motives; that means you should gather all the hard evidence as much as possible.

Keep everything from emails she sends you and record every interaction you may ever have had. You might also gather statements from witnesses. Save her text messages, record the conversation every time she calls, and gather them as possible evidence. You should also consider hiring a lawyer, especially when there is a divorce involved. Remember that things can get messy when dealing with this type of extreme narcissist.

Major Types of Narcissists and Their Subtypes

We have gone over the details of extreme narcissists in the previous section. Just to be clear, we're not saying that all narcissists are like that—

extreme. As stated earlier, the manifestations of this Narcissistic Personality Disorder vary from one person to another. It's just that there are some who are a little bit extreme.

Experts classify narcissists into three major types and under five common subtypes. Researchers have made distinctions between each type and they have also identified how these different types and subtypes can and do relate to one another. Let's begin with the three major types of narcissists and provide examples of each. As before, names have been changed to protect the identities of the women who have been generous enough to share their stories.

1. The Classic Narcissist

The classic narcissist is also called the grandiose narcissist. They are also known by other names such as exhibitionist narcissists and also as high-functioning narcissists.

When people describe a narcissist, this is the one that they are most likely be talking about. These are the attention-seekers and they love it when people flatter them. They want to be the focus of a conversation and often will hijack one just to have the limelight moved in their direction.

Notice how they get bored of a conversation if it isn't about anything that they are good at. The irony of it all is that in spite of this show of force, they are really vulnerable within. They want to feel important because deep down they feel worthless. They want to appear before others as superior because they feel inferior without that sort of perception of them.

Take, as an example, Miranda's mother:

"For as long as I can remember, my mom has loved being the center of attention. In preschool through freshman year of high school, I took ballet because she did it when she was that age. Whenever I had a recital, complete strangers would come up afterwards to compliment me on how well I had done, how graceful I was, and how beautiful I looked. Every time, without fail, my mother would divert the conversation to herself by saying something like, 'Oh, she gets it from me', 'I taught her

everything she knows' or 'She modeled that look after an outfit I wore for one of my recitals when I was her age. She's always telling me that she wants to be just like her mom'. Sometimes we'd stay for over half an hour after the recitals just so my mom could soak in the praise, even if I had homework to get done or if I was getting tired or hungry.

When I entered high school, though, I decided to pursue modern dance instead of ballet. It's a specific niche, and my mom knew nothing about it. Like with my ballet recitals, people would approach me after my modern dance recitals to congratulate me, but my mom would always act bored and insist that we had to get home so I could do my homework or that she was hungry or some other excuse. Any time the subject came up, she either got bored with it or diverted it back to my days dancing in the ballet—more specifically, how great SHE had made me at it."

Miranda's mother always made sure she was the center of attention, even if the conversation started off being about her daughter. She made sure that any praise Miranda got was redirected to her. Once Miranda got an interest/talent that her mother knew nothing about and had nothing to do with, she got bored with all conversations about it and even tried to turn them back to compliments about herself. Miranda's mother is a classic narcissist.

2. Vulnerable Narcissists

Although they crave being superior to other people, the vulnerable narcissist is not one that looks for the spotlight. They often become friends with those who are powerful and influential; they ride along on the wings of others.

But don't mistake it for weakness. It is all a covert maneuver to disguise their true nature. That is why narcissists of this type are also called closet narcissists, compensatory narcissists, and fragile narcissists.

They have a variety of tools at their disposal. At one point, they may assume superiority when needed. But then they also use a show of weakness to solicit pity and attention, thus gaining special treatment from others. At times, they do favors for others and will be exceedingly generous to them to ingratiate them. That is how they manipulate them and gain a big boost to their own self-worth.

Let's look at the case of Amanda's mother:

> *"None of us could really tell that mine and Mom's relationship was messed up for a long while. She just seemed like your typical doting mother. She would always get really worried when I was sick, crying and saying things like 'I don't know what I'd do if something happened to my baby!' It was understandable, especially when I was diagnosed with leukemia as a little kid and we were waiting for a bone marrow match (which fortunately came from one of my brothers). But it also happened for less severe sicknesses. She would tone it down when it was just something like a*

cold, but the message was still the same: pity me. Not pity my child, pity ME because MY child is sick.

Then, when I was in high school, I started dating the son of a really influential local politician. Mom was really nice and doing favors not only for me and my boyfriend but also for my boyfriend's father. I didn't think anything of it at first, just assuming that she was being nice, but then I noticed that everything nice she was doing for me was specifically in front of my boyfriend and his father. Then I saw her starting to do things like helping with my boyfriend's father's campaign, even though she had never been political before. He started to call her an 'angel' and a 'saint', even going so far as to call her a 'poor, modern-day martyr' when she told him about everything she had gone through when I was sick.

When I realized my boyfriend was emotionally abusing me, I tried to leave him, but my mother pressured me to stay with him as a favor to him and his father. She told me that my boyfriend really wasn't a bad guy, that he just needed a gentle hand and some help with his temper. She said that she was worried that I would be making a mistake that would make me miserable later if I didn't give him a chance, and I believed her. I ended up staying in that relationship for another two years before getting out, by the end of which I was a wreck and didn't trust anyone anymore. And after all that, I was the villain, and my now ex-boyfriend's father praised my mother for 'being the wonderful woman for assuring [his] son's happiness for even that long'."

It took Amanda a long time to realize that her mother was a narcissist because she never seemed like one. Everything she did either showed a vulnerable side to her—the "doting mother"—or seemed to be done out of the kindness of her heart for others. Even forcing her daughter to stay in a bad relationship was supposedly done out of concern for everyone else's happiness. As her mother was a vulnerable narcissist, Amanda didn't notice the signs until a lot of damage by both her mother and another emotional abuser had been done.

3. Toxic or Malignant Narcissists

Malignant or toxic narcissists are the types that exploit and manipulate others. The worst kinds of them have antisocial traits as well. In fact, experts often compare them to sociopaths or even to psychopaths.

Needless to say, these are the types of narcissists that you should stay away from. They manage, control, and lead the worst kinds of people in the world. Some of them even have a sadistic streak about them.

In their dealings with others, they only seek to dominate and control. At times, they will use aggression to gain control of other folks and, at times, they will use deceit. One common thread among people of this type is that they lack remorse for whatever wrong they may ever commit. The worst kinds of malignant narcissists even enjoy seeing other people suffer.

Terri had the misfortune of growing up with a malignant narcissist for a mother:

"Mother is one of the most manipulative people I've ever known. She turned me against my own father, her ex-husband, telling me that if I loved him, then I obviously couldn't love her. When I tried to console her and tell her that wasn't true, she told me that my father didn't love me, he just wanted me to spend time at his house so that she would be alone. She always said things to tear down my confidence, like my new shirt made my stomach bulge, I'd never get to a good school with my grades (usually B's) or that this or that friend only hung out with me because I had a car. The straw that broke the camel's back was when I was getting ready to interview for an internship at a huge tech company at nineteen and my mother told me that if they did hire me, it

would only be because my outfit was slutty and they thought I'd be easy.

After that, I finally took the steps to leave my mother and, to my surprise, my father took me in even though we hadn't spoken in years. It turned out that everything she had ever insulted me for were all insecurities she had had for as long as my father had known her, and the biggest reason they had gotten divorced was because she was always manipulating him and playing their friends and family members against him in order to get her way. That's when I realized she had done the same with me, and she had only kept me around so that she could use me to make my father miserable and insult me so that she'd feel better about herself. Worst of all, when I confronted her about it, she didn't feel at all guilty about it."

Terri's mother not only used Terri as a way to make herself look better but to also make sure that her ex-husband felt worse. She had been doing it her whole life, according to her ex-husband, but it seems that her poor daughter got the worst of it. I'd argue that Terri's mother is not just a malignant narcissist but possibly a psychopath.

Five Narcissist Subtypes

Sociologist Dr. Kristen Milstead has identified five subtypes of the three major types of narcissists. They include the following:

- Overt narcissists

- Covert narcissists

- Somatic narcissists

- Cerebral narcissists

- Inverted narcissists

The first two subtypes refer to the methodologies preferred by a narcissist to obtain control. An overt narcissist will be the one that is more open to the public and enjoys the spotlight. The covert narcissist subtype, on the other hand, is the one that will do their thing in the sidelines. They prefer to work their way in secret, using stealthy means to control and manipulate others.

You can say that covert narcissists are more passive-aggressive and overt narcissists are openly aggressive people. Given these two subtypes, we can therefore infer that classic narcissists will always belong to the overt subtype while vulnerable narcissists will always belong to the covert subtype. Note, however, that malignant narcissists can belong to either or both of the first two subtypes.

The next two subtypes refer to the things that the narcissist values the most. A somatic narcissist will put a huge value on their good looks and on their body. They are obsessed with their beauty, their appearance, and the things that they own, especially those that add to the value of their physical appearance.

A cerebral narcissist, on the other hand, is one that only values their intellect and being in control or being able to manipulate others, especially a crowd. Cerebral narcissists are the know-it-alls. They take pride in being able to bedazzle others with their intellect. That is how they obtain their position of power in any organization. Note that any of the three major types of narcissists can belong to any of these two latter sub types.

The inverted narcissist is a combination of the vulnerable and the covert types of narcissists. This is the type of narcissist that seeks the association and relationship with another narcissist.

They seem to be happy and content when they are in such a relationship. Some people call them as a victim-narcissist. They take the brunt of the pain and other abuse from their narcissistic partners, but they bask in the control and superiority of their narcissist partners.

Sometimes you can find them in husband-and-wife relationships. They raise their children under such tutelage, it is no wonder that some children end up emulating them. In other words, the child grows up to be a narcissist herself.

There is a common pattern that has been observed about inverted narcissist or victim narcissist. That is that they all suffered from abandonment issues when they were yet little children—

their father or maybe their mother left the family when they were still young.

How is NPD Diagnosed

If you're like I was, you'll probably try to get your mother to seek treatment before you do something drastic like cut contact with her—or, as was my case at the time, move out. If you are lucky enough to have a narcissistic mother who will be willing to undergo treatment, then please take every opportunity to bring her along to meet with a psychiatrist or other mental health worker.

If a loved one, a child, or some other sibling is showing the same signs or symptoms listed and described above, please take steps and consider early treatment. It should be noted that the symptoms of NPD are also similar to the symptoms of other personality disorders.

That is why it would be better to have a psychiatrist do the diagnosis. On top of that, it is also possible for one to be diagnosed with more than one type of personality disorder. Diagnosing NPD can be a bit challenging.

A psychiatrist's diagnosis will be based on several factors:

- The signs and symptoms that can be observed or have been observed about the person/patient

- Certain criteria that is based on DSM-5 or *Diagnostic and Statistical Manual of Mental Disorders*—a manual and comprehensive guide that is published by the American Psychiatric Association

- A thorough psych evaluation (the person being treated will be asked to fill out certain forms)

- A physical exam. Some physical and physiological issues are believed to be contributory to NPD. Part of the physical exam and diagnosis may include a CAT scan or some other brain scan.

What is the Treatment for NPD?

Psychotherapy is the treatment used today for Narcissistic Personality Disorder. It is basically a talk therapy and it has been found to be quite beneficial. Two of the main benefits that can be gained from this kind of treatment include:

1. An understanding of the causes of your emotions. You will know what actually drives you to despise yourself and others as well. You will also find out the deep-seated reasons that compel you to compete with others and what leads you not to trust other people, even those in your own family.

2. You will also learn how to better relate with other people. A person with NPD will learn how to build better relationships that are rewarding, enjoyable, and intimate.

Target Areas

The diagnosis and treatment procedures will help a person with narcissistic personality disorder to help accept certain realities and take responsibility for their actions. Some of the target areas include the following:

- Accept responsibility for and maintain personal relationships with coworkers

- Release any desire for goals that are utterly unattainable and unrealistic

- Learn to accept what one can really accomplish

- Learn to tolerate issues that relate to one's self-esteem along with the impact of such situations

- Learn to understand the feelings of others

- Obtain the power to regulate one's feelings

- Recognize which statements are criticisms and which ones are not

- Accept criticisms, tolerate them, and take responsibility for failures

The length of therapy will vary from one patient to the next. The severity of the symptoms will also have to be considered. Some therapy sessions can be short, which will be helpful to the patient when it comes to managing stress and crisis moments.

Some therapy and treatments can be provided on an ongoing basis. This will usually be provided after certain goals have been met. It also helps the patient maintain her own progress. Note that treatment will usually involve family members, friends, and anyone significant to the person being treated.

Medications for Treatment

There are no medications that will be recommended for people diagnosed with NPD. However, there may be related symptoms of other personality disorders or some other condition such as anxiety or depression.

For such conditions, your doctor may prescribe certain medications as part of your overall treatment. This will include anti-anxiety drugs as well as antidepressants, if they are warranted.

Possible Home Remedies

Home remedies for people diagnosed with NPD are given as part of the support for psychotherapy. Note that it is normal and quite common for such a person to be defensive and believe that such treatments are not really necessary.

They might even believe that such therapy is not worth the time. Be patient when trying to convince your narcissistic mother to go to therapy. In fact, she might only be convinced to go if you are willing to go there yourself.

Note that there will be many times when you will feel that you want to quit on your narcissistic mom. However, remember that it is important to keep an open mind and to keep your eyes on the prize, as it were. If you focus on the rewards of the treatment, then you will find hope that maybe your mother could get better and then you can start to have a real relationship with her.

Here are a couple more ideas that may help:

1. If there is a related drug or alcohol misuse along with the symptoms of NPD, then you should also get your mom treated for that as well. Addictions can feed off anxiety and depression and vice versa. This may also lead to a cycle of unhealthy behavior followed by emotional pain and back again.

2. Stick with the proposed treatment plan. If there are scheduled therapy sessions, then help your mom to attend those sessions. There will be setbacks and she will eventually try your patience. Is there anything new? She has already tried your patience many times over. So, why give up now when you are already moving in the right direction? Expect setbacks and plan your next moves when they happen.

What to Expect During Therapy Sessions

A psychiatrist or some other mental health provider will ask several probing questions. It may be more beneficial if your narcissistic mother is accompanied by someone she trusts or is on her good side. It could be her sister or brother or maybe your dad (her husband). Someone being there for her may help reinforce the treatment.

Your psychiatrist may also ask certain questions. It will help if you also think about these questions so you can help your mother along. Here are some of the most common questions your chosen psychiatrist may ask:

- Are you getting treatment for other medical conditions?

- Do you use alcohol?

- Do you do drugs?

- How often do you take alcohol/drugs?

- Have you ever been treated for any mental health issues in the past? If yes, then what treatments were effective for you?

- Do you have any relatives who have also been diagnosed with some other form of mental health illness?

- Describe your relationship with your parents?

- How do you feel when someone expresses their sadness to you?

- How do you feel when someone shows you that they are afraid?

- How do you feel when someone approaches you telling you that they are in desperate need of your help?

- What are your goals for the future?

- Please name your major accomplishments.

- Do you have any personal relationships with other people that you can say are close to you? Why or why not?

- How do you feel when someone criticizes you?

- What do you usually do to a critic?

- What symptoms are you showing?

- How do these symptoms affect your life and relationship to others?

- Do these emotions and thoughts affect your relationship with others at work, school, and at home? How do they affect these aspects of your life?

Keeping Realistic Expectations

Your psychiatrist (or other mental health provider) will try to find out possible underlying symptoms. They will also try to figure out the frequency of the symptoms and how they impact your life and your mother's life as well. However, your health worker might also come to the conclusion that somehow your mother might be beyond help. You should also prepare yourself for that eventuality.

I remember when I finally convinced my mother to come see a psychiatrist with me, I felt like I had a glimmer of hope. Even when we got there and I had to correct all my mother's false or fudged answers, I thought that there was at least hope so long as she was there with me. After a few sessions, though, it became clear that my mother was not going to cooperate. It came to the point that the psychiatrist told us flat out that she could not help us if my mother was not willing to actively and productively participate in her diagnosis and treatment.

It wasn't until later, when I was relating the story to my brother, that I said, "If she really loved me, she'd at least try," to which he replied, "Then we both know why she's not trying. For the same reason why she wouldn't try if I were the one in that shrink's office with her."

That's when I realized that he was right: no matter what I did, if she didn't care about me and didn't want to change, then she wouldn't.

And that might be the truth that you'll have to face with your own mother.

Chapter 5: Seven Essentials You Need Now as an Adult

A daughter of a narcissistic mother is an unloved daughter. She has never really had a mother all her life. Although every story of every daughter who has gone under such an abuse is unique, they often have commonalities that we can draw from.

One of the most common things that all daughters who have experienced narcissistic abuse is the fact they will eventually share the same needs as an adult. Understanding these needs and seeing the roles they play will help facilitate your healing.

Some of these needs you will perceive consciously. However, the daughter might fail to put them in the right context; that is, in the light of their childhood experiences. Unfortunately for some women, the recognition of traumatic effects of these experiences only occurs when she has grown older and when she is already living a life of her own.

However, for some, their adulthood brings a sense of newness. They feel that there are opportunities placed before them that weren't given to them when they were younger. Nevertheless, it doesn't matter if your new point of view is either bleak or hopeful. You still fail to see the huge emotional baggage that you have been carrying since your childhood.

What Prevents Daughters from Seeing the Truth?

There are several things that prevent a daughter from seeing or at least acknowledging that the childhood they experienced wasn't really normal. Chances are they still couldn't see its effects on their lives as an adult.

Somehow, someway, a daughter has pushed that cognition into her unconscious. There are other factors that prevent daughters of narcissistic mothers from getting that revelatory experience.

Here are some of them:

- You made your childhood experiences seem normal and justified them in your mind even though you felt that there was something wrong.

- You have alternated denial of the truth and hope for approval all through your life.

- You cling on to that desire more than anything for your mother to love you.

- You're afraid that maybe the way your mother treated you was really justified and that everything bad that happened to you was actually your fault.

- You want your childhood to be the same as everyone else's and, along with that, you are ashamed of your actual childhood experiences.

- You're still not ready to face the reality of your upbringing as a child.

- You prefer to think that the past is already over and that you are ready to move on— except that your past still haunts you to this day.

- You've been traumatized enough to block out the worst of the experiences.

What Makes an Abused Daughter Recognize and Acknowledge Reality

So, what would make a daughter of a narcissistic mother acknowledge the truth of her upbringing? It is more of a path to self-discovery, really. A lot of times, it comes along during therapy. That is why we recommend that you visit a therapist and hold regular sessions.

Sometimes, women go into therapy for a different reason. They feel unhappy, they have gone through a failed relationship, or maybe they have difficulty realizing their goals, etc. However, during the session, they will seem surprised that their current state of mind has something to do with their childhood.

That is how she rediscovers the root of her problems. Sometimes that discovery doesn't happen in therapy. Sometimes it comes from a loving friend who is honest enough to point it out to her. Sometimes that realization happens after a life-changing event in her life—like having a daughter of her own.

That can be quite an awakening because she of all people will not want her darling daughter to go through the same horrific experiences that she went through as a child. She might fear that she has already become like her narcissistic mother and has repeated the same pattern of abuse and pain.

For some women, the reality comes when they see their narcissistic mother verbally abuse her grandchild. That motherly protective nature sets in and she protects her child from the narcissist. It could be anger or it could be anything, but all she wants to do now is to protect her offspring, and she pushes all the denial and justification aside for the sake of her child.

Someone wisely pointed out that it is all about a woman's readiness to accept the truth. When she's ready to accept the truth, she will see and acknowledge the painful reality of the narcissistic abuse she went through.

Essential Needs of the Unloved Daughter

No matter how narcissistic abuse has impacted a daughter, victims will usually have several needs in common when they grow up as adults. They have all been deprived of each of these essential needs—it's one of the commonalities in the threads of their lives.

These needs have been denied to her since childhood. As an adult, she still longs for those needs to be fulfilled. Paradoxically, they coexist and contradict whatever success she may have attained in her life. Acknowledging these needs and fulfilling them in one way or another (completely or not) will be a huge step towards healing for the unloved daughter of a narcissistic mother.

1. A mother's love

An unloved daughter may rationalize that somehow, in her bizarre way, the narcissistic mother loved her. Yet she knows deep down inside her that a mother's love was absent and upon realization she will acknowledge that fact many years later as an adult.

This is actually a primal need—one that is hard-wired into every human being. We are social creatures and the first person to arouse that sociality within us is our mother. This isn't a purely rational desire, it is emotional, and it is deeply rooted in our genes.

Unfortunately, this isn't a need that will be fulfilled completely. A grandmother or another relative might step in and try to give this kind of love but their love can never completely replace the love of a mother.

This void can be made smaller and the lack thereof might be shrunk down to size, but it still remains.

2. Confirmation of her changed life

Someone needs to confirm that her life has now changed, that things are better now. That confirmation can come from a friend, a loved one, but the deepest kind is when the daughter sits down and confirms it all to herself.

She can do it by writing in her journal. She can also get that personal confirmation from pictures of her life now. She can also gain that confirmation by learning to live in the moment—one way to do that is through mindfulness meditation, which we will cover later on.

3. She needs to make sense of her past

An unloved daughter of a narcissistic mother will feel the need to make sense of her past and effectively disconnect it from her present experience. One thing that makes it all difficult is the cultural shame that comes with it—admitting the fact that your mother never really loved you.

She needs to externalize the issues, separate her experiences, and get away from the conditioning that it was her fault. Again, we recommend therapy sessions to fully make sense of your past. You can also try reflecting on them and compartmentalize the experiences and realize that they are separate from you.

4. She will need emotional balance

Every unwanted daughter of a narcissistic mom tends to be emotionally unbalanced. They don't know how to manage their painful emotions that come to them from time to time. When she experiences an intense emotion or a stressful situation, she finds difficulty and can't adjust to it accordingly.

However, the good news is that there are exercises that you can do to help you regulate your emotional experiences. We'll cover that in the next chapter.

5. She needs to build her self-confidence

A daughter of a narcissistic mother may doubt her own achievements. She may already be an accomplished woman yet deep inside her, her self-confidence is nowhere close to being rock solid. One way to help you build your self-confidence is to do a life review where you recall all the successes you have done and achieved in your life. You can then follow it up with affirmations. One specific type of therapy that we would like to recommend is CBT, or cognitive behavioral therapy.

That may help you get centered and eventually help you build that inner strength you have in you all along. CBT is a huge topic in itself and will require a separate work.

6. She needs her thoughts, perceptions, and feelings validated

It is very easy for a child to internalize all the things that have been said to her. A daughter who is constantly mocked, gaslighted, belittled, and insulted will have a lot of insecurities. That makes them easy to manipulate. She will tend to shy from any confrontation. Some even feel very sensitive to any form of criticism.

Validation of her true worth, her feelings, and her thoughts and perceptions will come from well-meaning friends. It will come from family who will be willing to support her. It will also come from counseling as well.

7. A sense of belonging

This is one of the most basic needs of human beings, whether you were narcissistically abused or not. An unloved daughter of a narcissistic mother needs to feel that she belongs somewhere. You can reconnect with friends, family, and other people who love you. You can join support groups where there are people with whom you can identify.

There is a community of people out there who have been through the same difficult times. You might not know them personally, but they are there. You can reach out to them either in person or online. Remember that you are not alone and that you belong.

In the next section, we are going to look at the first steps you can take to heal yourself. And if you like what you've learned so far, or you've found benefit, feel free to leave a review on Amazon. I really appreciate it as your feedback means a lot to me.

Chapter 6: First Steps to Healing

Any kind of abuse is utterly painful. That is a fact that no one can deny, especially if you have suffered some yourself. Physical abuse leaves traces on the body. Some injuries may even be permanent.

However, there are some injuries from abuse that are deeper, and they can hurt us for a lifetime. Emotional and mental scars are just that. They are extremely painful and yet they leave no scars. They are utterly difficult to unravel.

Those are two of the lasting effects of narcissistic abuse. It's an experience that we wouldn't want our children to suffer and yet it happens to children around the world. It first robs you of your confidence. You lose that singular trust in yourself.

After that, it also robs you of your sense of self. You feel like you don't have your own identity. In extreme cases, the victims of narcissistic abuse lose their sanity. The mind games that narcissistic parents play can sometimes take their toll on the child's mind.

You end up questioning your own behavior. Then you also question your natural feelings. You feel isolated and alone with no visible role model to turn to. You are left to figure out a terribly confusing world.

Toxic Relationships

There is no doubt that narcissistic relationships are toxic relationships. If you get immersed in it, your connection with your intuition is lost. Your natural discernment can also get lost or at least numbed. You can lose your sense of family and you may even lose your friends—or be afraid to make friends.

You see, in such a relationship, your narcissistic mom becomes your abuser. The most common tactic of abusers is to isolate their victims. It's just like a lion hunting its prey. The best way to win is not by superiority in numbers but by isolating the target and then capturing it while it is unable to defend itself and there is no one to help.

A narcissistic relationship is one of the strangest things. You may be in a relationship with someone who is supposed to be close to you and loving you, but in that relationship you will always feel alone. You can even say you have never felt more alone than now when you have someone to love.

Step 1: Waking Up to the Truth

One of the first steps to freedom and healing is to realize this one truth—you are not even in a relationship. The day you realize that fact is the day you get a huge wake up call.

That is the day when you wake up from that toxic relationship. Unless you come to this realization, you are powerless. You will never want change unless you realize that there is something wrong in your relationship with your narcissistic mother.

Step 2: Creating a Safe Haven

You can never hope to recover from narcissistic abuse if you do not create that safe space or that safe haven where you can find yourself again. A safe haven can be a place where you can go to in order to heal and sometimes it can just be a state of mind where all the hurt and pain will never reach you.

Along with the realization that there is something wrong with your relationship with your narcissistic mother, you should also come to realize that you need to get out of that relationship.

You need to sever that contact completely if you really want to be healed.

For really young children, another adult must intervene. It can be the other parent or it can be a concerned relative. If there is evidence of abuse to the child, then the parents can be reported to the authorities.

If you are older and have been under the clutches of an abusive narcissistic mom, your next step after realizing that something is wrong is that realization that you have the power to leave that kind of toxic relationship.

Since it is assumed in this book that you are the daughter of a narcissistic mother, then know that you can leave. There is nothing that your mother can do to stop you. If you are old enough to support yourself, then take the next step.

Take courage. I know it's a plunge but if you take it, you will breathe clean free air, so to speak. You are taking the opportunity to start anew and eventually take control of your own life the way you should have been doing it many years ago.

You can live alone, or you can live with someone else—someone who treats you as a person. It could be a relative. It could be a friend. But make sure that you will be living away from your narcissistic mom and living with someone you can trust.

Step 3: Creating an Inner Safe Haven

Sometimes you just can't leave. Whether you can leave or not, you can create what is called an inner safe haven. Maybe you're still too afraid to strike out on the world on your own. Maybe you are still anxious and afraid of what the world holds for you.

Maybe you are afraid of trying, and then failing, and then coming back to your narcissistic mother, which of course means you will incur her wrath. Sure, she'll take you back, but you will be in a worse condition than before.

If you cannot sever physical contact, then you can create a safe haven within. I'm talking about your emotions. That means when you interact with your abusive narcissistic mother, you should be able to separate your emotions from your person.

Remember that your emotions are part of you, but they are not you. You are not your emotions. Next time you interact or talk with your narcissistic mother, do not show any emotion or immediate reaction.

She humiliates you, then act as if you're bored. Act as if whatever she is saying or doing is not amusing. Do not fight back—that's exactly what your narcissistic mother wants. Don't fight back unless you are ready.

Doing that asks a lot from you. You will hear all the nasty things, all the insults and all the mean things she can say and do but you will have to bear it. Hold it all in. After the hell storm of words is over, ask to be dismissed or just simply leave.

Find some place where you can be alone. It can be in your car or it can be in your backyard. It can even be in the gym with your buddies. It can be at the beach. The important thing is that you have a place where you can be alone.

What do you do when you're all alone?

It's time to scream. Let all your frustrations out. If you're at the gym, then you can let all the steam out and try hitting a heavy bag. You can throw rocks at the ocean waves, yell at the trees. It's all up to you. What is important is that you have now found an outlet to let all your frustrations, angers, fears, and bottled-up emotions out.

After letting it all out, you will feel something different about yourself.

You have just learned to let go.

You have just let go of a lot of emotional baggage. Think about it. If you can let go of that, then certainly you can let go of a bad relationship, especially one that entails narcissistic abuse.

Once you have realized that you had it in you all along, you have already created a safe space within you. If words have no power to hurt you, then they have no power to control you. You are safe.

Step 4: Use the Power of Externalization

The next step is the big leap. Some people may be eager to begin a new life after realizing that they can choose to do so. However, you need to unload all the toxicity out of your life first before you can move forward.

Not only do you have to flush out all that toxicity that has been hedged up against you through all these years, you also need to relearn some things—like learning to love yourself for who you are.

Here are a few suggestions that will help you facilitate the purging of all that toxicity. These techniques have been dubbed as externalization (i.e. the opposite of internalizing things).

- **Be on the move**

When you are hurting, it is easy to just want to mope about it or stay at home and feel sorry for yourself. Sulking is such an attractive option because it's easy. All you have to do is stay in bed all day. Eat everything that's there in the fridge and live life as a couch potato.

It's important that you get out of bed and maybe get out of the house. Studies have shown that people who exercise for at least 2 hours each week will become less prone to depression compared to folks who live sedentary lives.

However, do take note that it's okay to feel sad for all the bad experiences that you had with your narcissistic mom. So, go ahead and take your time to grieve. However, you should also take time to go out and stretch a little.

Staying at home all day feeling sorry for yourself sets you up for depression. People who do that have a 44% risk of developing depression, as one study pointed out. You can start by stretching.

Well, that way you don't have to go out of the house just yet. You can also try some yoga. If you have a treadmill, then use that. Just 15-30 minutes of exercise each day will give you outstanding benefits.

It doesn't even have to be some fitness program or something like that. You can even just find a music video and dance to it. The important thing is that you are moving and you are exercising and that you are enjoying whatever it is you're doing.

- **Walk**

Make it a habit to have 15 to 30 minutes of exercise. After that, you can take the next step—walking. Put on your headphones, play your favorite music, and walk around the block.

Exercising is great but, you see, you're still in a confined space. That confinement can play tricks on your mind. After a week or so of staying at home, your thinking space can get a little too crowded. So, the solution is to expand your thinking space—get out of the house and see the world.

I suggest that when you go out to walk; do it where you can get in touch with nature like in a park or some nearby woods. Nature is a great healer of emotions. Being in nature will help reduce stress, fear, and anger. It will also increase your good feelings and boost your physical well-being.

I also suggest that you go for a walk in places where you can be alone with your mind. Remember, you're trying to expand your thinking space, right?

Now, here's another tip—walk and then give yourself some positive self-talk. Talk to yourself while you're at it. Let all your frustrations out. Then look around you and see the wonders of Mother Nature.

There is a huge body of evidence that supports the fact that exercise and walking in particular can help ease depression and sadness. One BBC news report drew its sources from medical reviews and reported that going for a brisk stroll can play a significant role in keeping depression away.

On top of that, walking while talking to yourself is a great form of self-therapy. Talking to yourself and hearing your own voice can help to evoke compassion for the self.

At one point, you may find yourself breaking down and crying about it all over again. When that happens, then just let it all out. Let all the grief and sorrow get flushed away. But you should also notice that after the sorrow has been expressed, there is a loving universe out there and it is telling you that the life ahead of you is as wide as the expanse that is before you.

- **Use affirmations**

Use daily affirmations that you can tell yourself. You can do it first thing when you wake up. You can say them to yourself while you're brushing your teeth, looking at your reflection on the mirror.

You can purchase an affirmations book, but you don't really have to. You can even download an app for your phone where you can read or even hear the affirmations being spoken.

The important thing is that you listen deeply or read the text deeply. You can even record your own voice as you say these sample affirmations.

- I love myself.

- I'm a strong woman.

- I'm a survivor.

- I can tell my narcissistic mom that I'm done with her.

- I am a nice person, unlike my mother.

- I can take care of myself without my mother's help.

Again, this is another form of positive self-talk. It is something that you can keep telling yourself until you realize that you actually believed it in the first place. No one loves you more than you. There is something about hearing your own voice telling you things that you need to hear that heals you from within.

- **Write a journal**

Some have recommended that journaling should be made into a daily habit. It's a way to let out all the frustrations and the hurt that you experienced in your relationship with your narcissistic mother.

However, I suggest that if you do this, make sure to write your journal entries in such a way as if you will want someone to read it some-time in the not-so-distant future. Write your entries as if what you have penned down on those pages will be a great benefit to someone who may also be suffering the same things that you have suffered.

Write them as if you are reaching out and giving hope to someone else. You will never know who might read it in the years to come. It could be your son, your grandchildren, and, who knows, it might just be you reading your entries in the coming months.

Your journal is going to work like a time capsule. The pain and hurt you felt will catch up to you from time to time. But when they do, you can always go back to your journal and read about how you found hope in spite of the pain. Take the advice that you gave to yourself many months or years ago. Then see how much you have grown and how far you have gone.

Writing is a good introduction to meditation. If you have just come out of a traumatic experience, your thoughts will be out of whack. The memories of your pain will come flooding into your mind, which might sometimes hinder you from properly meditating.

Writing things down can slow things down for you. Remember that the pen is slower than the mind. That way, you can focus on one life event at a time. Journaling also has proprioceptive benefits. It can help your brain access some old memories that you have locked away. It's a chance to unwind and dump all the hurt and finally make it all exit your soul.

- **Reach out**

There are support groups for people who were raised by narcissists; believe it or not, joining them and voicing your story will help. Support groups are, again, safe spaces. It's a place where you can voice all the drama that you ever had at home. The big difference is that this time there are people who are willing to listen and they do care.

If you don't think that you can face a group of people just yet, even though they are people like you who also suffered narcissistic abuse, then just try it once. You are still voicing your story and you are still reaching out. Yes, there are online support groups for children raised by narcissist mothers.

One such group is the raisedbynarcissists Reddit group. There you can post your grievances, your thoughts, and your experience. You can also read about the experiences and the issues that other children like you have gone through.

If you're interested, you can start now by underline clicking here.
[https://www.reddit.com/r/raisedbynarcissists]

- **Try new things**

Trying out something new is part of your huge leap into healing. It instantly switches you from processing your terrible experiences in the past to looking forward to a new, exciting, and different experience.

It's easy. Write down all the things that you always wanted to do and try but couldn't because of your previous experience with your narcissistic mother. Make that into a to-do list or a bucket list of sorts.

Your list could be anything like try Japanese food, go skiing, take a spa break, buy those clothes, get that toy, talk to your crush, write a book, and a lot of other things. As long as it is something you haven't done before, put it in your list.

Now, pick one item in your list and work on it. Keep trying until you get the courage to actually do it (like talk to your crush?). Some of the things on your list might take some time (paint a picture?), so you can do that on some days and then pick another task that is easier to do (getting some pampering in a spa?) so that you have a short-term goal achieved and a long-term goal in the works.

Studies have shown that when we try something new, we are moving ourselves to new environments and new experiences. It enhances our mindfulness (more of that later). In effect, you shift your brain's activity from focusing on past hurt to new things that excite you, thus creating new neural pathways. Soon, you realize that the doors have been swung open and you are now beginning to live a new life.

- **Record everything and share them online**

Making an online record is an extra step, you can do it if you want or you can just skip this step. However, just note that there is a benefit to recording your experiences in video, text, or voice. Recording, as it has been found, helps to depersonalize any kind of traumatic experience.

It externalizes the experience and allows you to see it from a third-person point of view. It eventually helps to broaden perspective. At one point, you will grow a certain level of compassion towards others, realizing that you are not the only one in the world to ever suffer from abuse—narcissistic or otherwise.

Note that these are only the first few steps to healing and recovery from a narcissistic relationship. We will go over the other things that you can do in order to sustain whatever progress you may already have achieved.

Chapter 7: Understanding and Overcoming Grief

There are two overwhelming emotions that stir you up inside after going through narcissistic abuse—grief and anger. Note that both these emotions have their place when it comes to your complete recovery. They are very natural reactions to any form of traumatic experience. In this chapter, we'll go over what grief is and its place in the recovery process. We will deal with the other emotion, anger, in a separate chapter.

Grieving for the Mother You Never Had

One of the things that you need to get over as a daughter of a narcissistic mother is mourning for the things that you never had, things like support, love, and genuine interactions that you missed out on when you were a child.

You never really had genuine laughter with your narcissistic mom because when she laughed with you, she had something else in mind—an ulterior motive behind it all. She never really got attuned to you.

Grieving allows you to feel. It helps you to let go of the labels that were branded upon you. It can also help you to let go of that paralyzing fear that maybe there is no one out there who will love you.

Allow yourself to weep for the mother that you deserved and never had. Some have said that screaming, yelling, hitting the bed and the pillows in rage and anguish doesn't really help the anger. That is true—doing those violent things doesn't make the anger go away.

But—and that is a big but there—doing all that allows you to get in touch once again with your feelings. You get to realize that you are an individual and not just an extension or a tool of your narcissistic mother. You are your own person because you can feel yourself getting angry and you are grieving for something that is totally for yourself.

The Stages of Grieving

Research today had acknowledged and identified the 5 specific stages of grief that adult children of narcissistic mothers go through.

These stages don't necessarily have to be experienced in any order. In fact, some stages overlap with others as one goes through them. Let's go over each of these five stages in the discussion below:

- **Acceptance**

One stage of a grieving daughter is acceptance. She learns to accept that her narcissistic mother really had very minimal love for her. On top of that, she learns to accept that her mother didn't really have any capacity for empathy.

She also learns that she cannot allow herself to continue to live in denial. Through acceptance, she learns to acknowledge her feelings again. Acceptance is actually the next step in the recovery process after one realizes and acknowledges that there is a problem in one's relationship with one's narcissistic mother.

• **Depression**

When a daughter accepts the fact that she never really had a true loving relationship with her mother, she will eventually feel a certain level of depression. The truth comes crashing down.

She feels an intense sadness. On the one hand, she has accepted the fact that she has to let go of the last slivers of hope that she will one day have that loving relationship she envisions with her mother. Remember that the effect of a narcissistic mother is stronger on a daughter than with a son.

She impacts the daughter so powerfully simply because she should have been the role model that the daughter was supposed to emulate. The daughter will eventually realize that her mother will never be as loving as she thought she could be.

She will see the love she never had in the relationships she observes in her friends and their mothers. She will envy what she could never have. In effect, she will feel like an orphaned girl even though she is living in a home with her parents in there.

She will let go of all those expectations. She will feel the onset of depression. Along that line, she will also feel anger and grief creep in as well.

- **Bargaining**

The daughter of a narcissistic mother has been bargaining for her mom's love and affection all her life. They do their bargaining internally as well as with her mother. Inwardly, she will have a very common dialogue with herself.

She will say, "If only I can become good enough, then my mom would love me." She will do all sorts of bargaining from making good grades, being polite, being kind, being obedient, and others.

At one point, she will talk to her mother and will bargain with her. She will offer to do one thing and hope that she can plea bargain going out for ice cream or something. Sometimes it works, but most of the time, Mother just won't be bothered— or she just doesn't want to bother with her daughter.

During all of this, realities tend to get confusing as she contrasts what she sees in other kids with the experience she's been having. Sometimes even after a daughter has been separated from her narcissistic mother, she may still be bargaining within her just to deny the reality that she is now trying to cope with.

I spent a lot of time in this particular stage of the grieving process. I thought for sure that if I were different, if I were better, that things would get better between my mother and me. Maybe, I thought, I could get her to see that what she was doing was wrong. It can happen—the problem is that I spent more time than I should have on trying to make it work. I did all the work while my mother didn't even promise to try to be better.

Even after I consciously realized it wouldn't work and went to live with my brother, deep down, I still told myself, "Maybe if I just make the effort to reach out first, she'll be touched enough to compromise." I was just lucky that my brother served as a reality-check for me and helped me realize that no matter how much I bargained, it wouldn't get me our mother's love.

• Anger

Another stage in the grieving process is anger. Believe it or not, this is a necessary step in order for one to recover from it all. A daughter will feel anger for her mother because she didn't get her emotional needs met.

She will get angry at the fact that all the hope she had that her mother would change has been crushed by nothing short of the truth. One would feel anger towards the parent for doing all the harmful things she has done and also towards oneself for allowing such things to happen.

Being angry is a stage when one feels stuck. No matter what you do, however, you might lash out in anger at the world, nothing satisfies your rage. How do you get over that? We'll cover that in the next chapter.

• Denial

As a child, the young daughter has been denying the facts to herself and to others. She denies certain truths that she really knew all along such as her mother doesn't really love her, and she denies that her mother couldn't show empathy.

Why do the children of narcissistic mothers deny the truth? They do it in order to survive. The child yearns for love above everything else that she has been given or will ever receive. She denies the truth in order to grow, and she does it even when faced with cognitive dissonance.

Overcoming Grief

While she's in the grieving process, the daughter of a narcissistic mother will shift from one phase to the next until eventually she learns to let go. Here is a step-by-step process that will help that daughter overcome grief.

1. *Be patient with oneself*

Being patient with yourself will buy you enough time to accept what really happened between you and your narcissistic mother. Do not give yourself any schedule, there are no deadlines. In fact, just allow the emotions to come and go as they please. Later on, we'll go over mindfulness techniques and exercises to help you cope with the flood of emotions that come at you.

At this point, remember that all you are trying to do is to overcome the grief you are feeling. Doing so will require a lot of patience. You will feel sorrow, you will feel self-pity. Everything that has a beginning, which includes this grief and sorrow that you feel, everything, has an ending. Your grief will begin and one day it will end and be gone permanently.

2. Learn to adjust your expectations

After being patient with yourself for a while, you will come to a point when you can accept the fact that the loneliness that you are feeling now is just part of the grieving process. Sorrow is natural and so are the other emotions that you will feel, including hate, anger, and regret.

Once you have come to the point that you already accept the truth that your narcissistic mother had very little love and care for you, you can now adjust your expectations. Make adjustments in your expectations of your mother and of yourself.

Note that your experience will not be linear. You won't go from grief to anger to resolution and then finally to new life. It doesn't work that way. You will at one point overcome sadness and start rebuilding your life. You may be trying something new like a new career path but then comes one or two triggers.

They trigger your memories and you then feel anxiety and grief all over again. Sometimes you will question yourself—"I thought I was over this?"

Again, adjust your expectations. Things like that tend to come back to haunt you from time to time. Since you now expect all the hurt, anger, and grief to come back, you should plan for it.

Find your safe place—it can be in the company of friends or it can be in a fortress of solitude in your very own mind. You can stack up and build mental fortitude, but it will take time. It puts us back again to step 1—be patient with yourself. Remember that these steps aren't linear, either. You are free to skip from one step to the other and come back as needed.

3. *Learn to accept all the things that you can never change*

Again, this third step can be transitioned from step 3 to step 1 or even step 2. In fact, you can move this step anywhere along the way. Again, there is not a linear way to do it when it comes to processing your grief.

However, coming to accept the things that you cannot change is a crucial part of the process on how to overcome grief. This is actually a key step.

As a daughter of a narcissistic mother, you may feel that everything is out of your hands. You feel that you have no control over a lot of things—or maybe you can't control anything.

Of course, that is not true. You have a choice and you can control a lot of the aspects of your life. You can choose not to be angry when someone makes a disparaging remark. You can choose to believe in one person over another. You can even choose what to wear for your coming date. You can choose which color of lipstick you want to put on.

However, along with that realization that you have control, you should also come to terms with the things that you can't change. For example, you have to learn to accept that you can't change your mother. No matter how much good you do and how much you forgive and reach out to her, she may already be out of reach. You may no longer have any influence on her to make the necessary change.

There is no point in fixing and gluing together the proverbial broken mirror. You might even end up cutting yourself in the process. Even if you were able to put all the pieces back together, the image you get from the mirror is already broken and will never be whole again.

4. Find strength in people

If it weren't for two people, I probably would not have found the strength to accept the fact that I could not change my mother and had to move on with my life: my brother and my paternal grandmother.

For the longest time, my brother was the only one to see our mother for who she is, an abusive narcissist. Even our father remains in denial. My brother did everything he could to convince me that our mother was horrible to us, but I thought I could change her. He never gave up on me, and when I finally came around, he helped me get out of there and even gave me a place to stay.

After that, my paternal grandmother served as the mother I never had. She believed what my brother and I told her about our mother—even believing us over her own son—and comforted us both. She served as a safe, nonjudgmental person to go to while we grappled with the emotional scars our mother had left on us. And they are just two of the many friends and family members who helped me during this time.

One of the tactics used by abusive people is to isolate their victims—we already mentioned this earlier. This isolation actually cuts you off from any potential support system that you would have benefited from while the abuse was ongoing.

You can get that much-needed support from anyone that cares. They don't even have to say anything, and all they need is to care enough to listen to you. Yes, that may sound like you are using them as a sounding board, but that isn't really asking much.

A friend who will lend a listening ear does more to help you than a relative or a minister in church who is more interested in giving you a piece of his mind. In effect, when they listen to you, they are actually lending their strength, albeit a small portion of that strength.

Small or not, that strength that you draw from their patience and empathy will go a long way. They don't necessarily have to be people who have gone through the same experience as you have; as long as they can empathize, then you're good to go.

You see, for most of her life, the daughter of a narcissistic mother has never had someone empathize with her. It would be helpful for her to have a good female role model that she can look up to. That woman could be an aunt, a family friend, a coworker, a teacher, the mom of her friend, and others.

It will help her not only to survive through the situation but to thrive in life through the years to come. Having that someone who can feel her pain is a much-needed change and can help to facilitate the release of the feelings of grief.

5. *Don't get stuck both literally and figuratively*

Take this piece of advice seriously—don't get stuck.

Don't get stuck in the house day after day. That will just feed your grief. Don't get stuck on the feelings of anger and frustration that you have in there. Let them out. Let yourself out of the door, too.

Go out. Go somewhere new. Try something new.

Talk to your doctor. Go schedule an appointment with your therapist. Find a new hobby. Adding more new experiences to your life will help you find that meaning that you may have lost while you were in isolation with a narcissistic parent.

This is a time when having a strong support system could really help you. Friends and family will give you space when you need it, but if it seems like you're getting stuck, they're one of the best sources for setting a fire under you. Let them know that you want to get out and try new things, that you're looking for a therapist or even that you don't want to spend more than X days in a row without leaving your house. They'll help you in any way they can, even if that means "kidnapping" you for lunch at that new deli by Grandma's house (much like my brother did under my paternal grandmother's instructions).

6. *Make plans and make use of your time*

Realize that time is like money. It is some form of emotional and mental currency. Just like money, there will always be time. You don't run out of money—if you lose some, then you can surely earn some along the way.

The same is true with time. You can choose to spend it wisely now or you can just keep on waiting to spend it on a day that will never come. You won't be here forever, but there will always be time that you can spend each day of your life. Spend it well and stop dwelling in the past.

7. *Create value from your experiences*

Every experience is a learning point in your life. As you reflect on your experience with your narcissistic mother, other than focusing on the hurt and pain, why not look for life lessons in them instead?

When an awful experience comes to mind again, try to look at it from another perspective. Find something that you can learn from. Treat it like reading a book. Sure, you have gone over it time and again. But just like any book, you can find more threads of faith that you can learn from.

8. *Celebrate life*

It's a tragic injustice if you are left trapped focusing on the loss and pain that you experienced with your narcissistic mother. Staying in that state doesn't help you move on and it doesn't help you heal.

An alternative that you can choose is to celebrate life—a new lease on life that you now have in your hands. The past is now over and it's time to move on. Someone once said that we can't do anything about the past other than accept it. The future isn't exactly ours since we can't predict it. The only time you have control over is now.

My current therapist keeps a clipping of a 1994 "The Family Circus" cartoon strip by Bil Keane taped to the back of her laptop, and under the drawing, it reads, "Yesterday's the past, tomorrow's a mystery, but today is a GIFT. That is why it's called the present." It might be a bit cheesy, but whenever I start thinking about how my mother treated me and start questioning why I wasn't good enough, I think about this quote and decide instead to celebrate the now.

You need to live in the moment because this is all you know. There is no longer anyone pulling the strings. You have been freed, and there is an entire life waiting to be lived by no one else but you.

Chapter 8: Dealing with Anger

How do I stop being angry?

That must be a question that you have asked yourself a million times. You will be asking this question when you have arrived at the point in your life when you already understand what went on during your childhood.

You know and understand that you were a victim of an abusive relationship. You are angry at your narcissistic mother for treating you with cruelty instead of love. You will feel anger for your father who was passive or just absent. Sometimes you will come to realize that your father was an accomplice to all the abuse that you received at that time. You may even feel anger towards your brothers and sisters who just stood by and did nothing.

The anger you feel has its uses. On the one hand, it can help you understand the reality of the situation you were in. But on the other, continuously harboring all that anger will bring up more problems that you will have to deal with. It's something you just don't need at the time while you're still trying to recover.

Sometimes we hide behind a mask of anger. Well, it is certainly easier to hide behind a façade of toughness armed with a biting sarcastic quip whenever someone pries into your personal affairs.

It's certainly an easier mask to wear instead of the other one. What other mask? It's the one that shows that you are insecure, afraid, and vulnerable. Does that reaction sound familiar? Yes, it is the very same action or reaction that your narcissistic mother had—hiding behind the appearance of control and power but deep inside one is actually truly helpless.

At first, you wouldn't connect this anger you felt with your childhood experiences. That is pretty common—denying the truth of it all. However, after some self-evaluation and also some soul-searching, you will learn to accept the truth and know where all that anger is coming from.

Slow Recognition

The anger of a daughter raised by a narcissistic mother surfaces as soon as she realizes (and of course understands) why Mother treated her that way. She begins to know how her attitude and treatment affected her.

It takes a while before that happens. That realization is preceded by a sense of wrongness in the family. Even at a young age, she realizes that something is off, but she can't quite put a finger on it.

She would be in a state of denial. In effect, even though she is being maltreated, she will still think mother is doing it for her own good. She might even begin to wonder why she wasn't good enough. If there is a brother in the family, she may even begin to think that her brother had all the right checkmarks ticked off and she could barely get anything done right.

It will take a significant amount of time before she could put one and one together. Some women have already married or are already forging their careers when they finally find out and realize what happened.

Part of this slow recognition includes the fact that she coped with her situation in the hope that she would be able to fix things. She was hoping that she could somehow normalize her situation. She rationalized her mother's behavior and then dissociated the pain she felt. It's all in a confused effort to win her mother's love.

Two things collide in her world—her need for Mother's love that she so desperately wants and her growing recognition of the wrongs that are being committed. The effect, of course, is cognitive dissonance.

The Turning Point

The next question is what will stop a daughter's cognitive dissonance? The answer is simple—her growing recognition of what is really going on. Every cup that you fill slowly will tend to get filled up in the end—metaphorically speaking.

That is what happens to a child raised under the cruelty of a narcissistic mother. She gets fed up, so to speak. All the maltreatment that she received have all been stacked and piled high; well, in this case, it is already too high. She then switches from needing her mother's love to surviving her mother's version of "loving."

All the abuse flips her fight-or-flight switch. Unfortunately, this time the flight option has been virtually scratched off due to overuse. Now she is ready to fight back—anger at this point is a good thing. All the denial that she's been using has now been swept aside. Before this point, she was afraid of facing her mother and the reality of her situation—now she is ready for a confrontation.

It's Hardwired into Every Human Being

Believe it or not, human beings are actually hardwired for anger. It's one of our coping mechanisms. It is the emotion that we unleash when we want to get things done and fast. Experts call it the stress response.

Unfortunately, this fight-or-flight response is a double-edged sword. On the one hand, it powers you up to do what you might have not done otherwise. On the other, it is a state that numbs our ability to think straight.

Researchers have tested the effects of anger on human beings. Physiologically, you are pumped up. Your blood pressure rises, and you feel that hot flash that runs all over your body.

That's the physiological response. The next question is what happens in your head? Researchers ran MRIs on test subjects and tested their decision-making skills and lexical ability when they're angry and when they are not.

It has been confirmed that the response time to lexical triggers of human beings increase when they're angry. That means that the slightest words said to you can make you snap rather quickly. For instance, trigger words like the disparaging remarks used by your narcissistic mother can immediately trigger a violent response when you are angry.

That is a good thing for certain circumstances. However, researchers also found out that your decision-making skills and other high cognitive capabilities are reduced when you're angry. That means if you stay angry or keep repressed anger, for the longest time you may find yourself stuck in your situation.

You are no longer moving forward since you are fixated on the thing that made you angry. In other words, anger can prevent you from moving on with your life. It also prevents you from healing from narcissistic abuse.

It's Okay to Be Angry with Yourself

Some women who were daughters of narcissistic mothers feel shame and anger at themselves. They are angry for playing along with their mother's manipulative ways. Some berate themselves for being so stupid—their choice of adjective. That ultimately feeds their self-critical inner voice.

However, you should know that being angry at yourself is okay. It is a natural response. Now, the question is how you deal with it.

Anger in the Context of the Grieving Process

In the previous chapter, we described anger as part of the grieving process or one of the stages in our moments of grief. Anger in such a context has a place in our eventual recovery from abuse.

Anger allows you to feel or recognize your emotions and your individuality again. A daughter raised by a narcissistic mother at one point will feel that she has lost her individuality. She will think that she only serves certain purposes and that is to give joy and honor to her mother.

In such a situation, every good thing she does elevates her mother's status and stature. On the other hand, every time she does something wrong (acts impolitely or has a tantrum) then it brings shame and dishonor to her mum.

Anger releases tensions that are within you. All those excuses are brushed aside, and you immediately let the world know (your mother included) that you exist. You shout out and tell the world that you are a human being with needs that are waiting to be filled. Anger in this context is a self-preservative tool.

How Do You Deal with Anger

One of the ways to deal with anger is to work it out within the context of the grieving process. Remember that the grieving process as it was outlined in the previous chapter is an action plan for letting go.

If you go through the process, then you will learn how to let go of pain, disappointment, your frustrations, and, of course, your anger. One part of the process or phases is the acceptance that your mother will never change and that your relationship with her can never be salvaged. If that is the way it has to be concluded, then you just have to accept it for what it is.

Some narcissistic mothers can change, and some cannot. When push comes to shove and you find out that she will never change, then there is no point in hanging on. Letting go ends the core conflict and that ends the anger. Once the core issues have been let go, then there is no longer any reason to get angry.

Use Rituals for Letting Go

Here is Hannah's story:

"My mother was long gone and I was starting a family of my own. However, I still felt angry at myself for allowing my mother to dictate a huge portion of my life. You can say that I already lost my childhood and a portion of my adult life after being abused by a narcissist mother.

Right after I got married, my mother got sick and a few weeks after that she died. I was the only child and my father had passed away. The funeral was short and there weren't a lot of words to say, but the hurt still lingered several years after she was gone. As a memento, I kept her urn.

I found my healing when a friend suggested that I throw away her ashes into the sea. I thought that it was a great idea. I found that it was my own way of saying goodbye for good.

I also gathered up pictures and other things that reminded me of my painful childhood. It included clothes that she made me wear, pictures of me she took—there was never a picture of both of us together—and then there were other things.

All of that I burned, too, and put the ashes in a box. My husband and I went to the beach the following day. I scattered my mom's ashes into the sea along with the ashes of the things I burned.

The feeling of release I got from that was astounding. I was letting go, it was goodbye, and it was for good."

Rituals of mourning don't have to be as dramatic as that. You can create your own rituals where you can pour in your heart's desire. All your hate and anguish can be contained in that singular moment and then you let go and say goodbye for good.

Some daughters have written goodbye letters that they never intended to send. The letters contain all the details that they wanted to share with their mother that they knew their mothers wouldn't even bother to read or pay attention to anyway. Some letters were burned, and others were buried in the ground.

Believe it or not, my paternal grandmother had given me the idea rather than another survivor or a therapist. I had confided to her how mad I was with my mother for making me feel like I was never good enough, and she told me she had written this sort of letter to my grandfather after he died in a car accident. She was mad at him for driving drunk that night—and many other nights—and told me that the act of writing out all her emotions, even she couldn't tell him directly, made her feel better. Destroying it, she said, was almost more effective than writing it.

When I wrote mine, I used all the rage I had left to rip it up until the pieces were too small for me to rip up anymore and then dumped the pile into the trash. I have to admit, it felt pretty good to let all of those emotions out all at once, both in getting them out on paper and in getting rid of the letter.

Pour your heart out when you go over your ritual. Make it yours. Finally, say goodbye and let it all go. Walk away from it all and go forward in your new life.

Chapter 9: Detachment and Setting Boundaries

There are women who aren't so lucky. They are left with no other option but to continue interacting with a narcissistic mother. That means that the toxic interactions will continue. You might find it interesting that even though you have said goodbye to her, she will still find a way to poke her nose into your business from time to time.

I recommend a two-step process for dealing with such a situation. Here are the steps:

1. Detach with love

2. Set healthy boundaries

We'll go over these steps in the discussion below.

Detaching with Love

What is the one key characteristic that differentiates you the daughter and your narcissistic mother? That characteristic is empathy. It makes a whole world of a difference, especially when conflicts arise in your relationship with one another.

Whenever you clash with your mom, you care about every word said and that is why it hurts you deeply. Your mother, on the other hand, doesn't care. You tend to reach out trying to help her, she does not. You try to find reconciliation between you two, she does not.

If that doesn't drain you emotionally and mentally, then I don't know what will. So, what's the solution? It is to detach with love. To detach from someone is to separate from that person and to create space in between you two.

Again, that is an important part of healing from narcissistic abuse. But some people will have a hard time doing that, especially those daughters who are also high-level empaths. They will still have a place in their heart for Mother, which is why letting go is so difficult.

This is where detaching with love fits in nicely. It allows you to separate but still maintain some sort of emotional connection. It allows you to heal your own soul first and it also allows the other person (i.e. the one you are detaching from) to find time to find solutions for her own problems.

Randl Kreger used an interesting analogy to describe what detachment with love is like. It is spot on. It also shows us that we may have already been doing it in our day-to-day business as we interact with other people:

> *"If the world were a store and someone came up to you looking for the auto parts section, detaching would be like saying, 'I'm sorry, but I'm not the sales clerk. I don't know where the auto parts are; perhaps you can find a sales clerk at the customer service counter.' It's not saying, 'Let me find out for you,' and it's not snapping 'Do you see me wearing a uniform? No? Then leave me alone!'"*

Detaching with love is like saying no to your narcissistic mother, and you do it without investing any more emotions to the issues that she is raising. When she says all of that is your fault (or some other disparaging or hurtful statement), then you disengage from her emotionally and identify what she is doing. You've been through it before; you already know what her game plan is.

You can only detach with love when you have found your inner peace and emotional fortitude. If not, then your emotions will go all over the place. You will just engage her, and you feed her ego with your reactions.

You show her that you are not emotionally invested when you say no to her and act bored, as if the subject she is bringing up doesn't really concern you at all—and it doesn't.

Expect to get some resistance when you do this. Hang in there. The moment the narcissist notices that her antics no longer work, she will give up eventually. This takes practice, though, and a lot of patience. This way, you are giving compassion to your mother by not engaging her and you are showing compassion to yourself by not getting emotionally attached, thus allowing you to heal.

Setting Healthy Boundaries

This is a two-step process, right? After you have detached with love, the next thing you should setup are healthy boundaries with your mother. Now, just like the first step, you may have to repeat this process several times over until it sinks in. That is just how stubborn a person diagnosed with Narcissistic Personality Disorder will be.

Setting healthy boundaries includes putting up rules about your interactions with one another. They include rules on being rude, insults, privacy, disparaging remarks, and other forms of behavior—especially around your children. You don't want your narcissistic mother's toxicity to affect your own kids, too.

You can write down all the house rules if you like or you can just memorize them. This gives you and your mother some structure in your interactions so that everyone knows how far they can go.

Along with the rules that you are making comes consequences. Each time your narcissistic mom crosses the line, there should be a consequence. Remember that the rules also apply to you as well but expect your mother to break them more than you do. The consequence can be anything from not talking to her for a given number of hours to cutting off financial support.

Useful Tips for Talking to Narcissist Mothers

Here are 5 tips on how to set boundaries with a narcissistic mother:

1. *You should know where to draw the boundaries in your relationship*

When writing down the rules, you should decide which behaviors are acceptable and which ones are not. You should make these rules and boundaries clear. You will have to repeat them over and over until your narcissistic mom remembers them.

So, for instance, if you don't want any bullying, insults, and name calling, then make sure to state that they will never be tolerated. You can say something like this:

"If you continue to insult me, call me names, or bully your way, then this conversation is done. I will not speak to you until 5 o'clock this afternoon."

The consequence must be clear. It can be time-bound or not. But remember that it has to be conditional. In the example above, time is the condition. You can set other conditions as well such as "until you become respectful" or something to that effect.

Expect your mom to resist these rules and boundaries. She may even continue to berate you after making that spiel. However, you can enforce the boundary immediately. For instance, as in the example above, if your mom continues to insult you after setting your boundaries, you should immediately give her the cold shoulder. You literally don't have to talk to her, which, of course, enforces the penalty you mentioned earlier.

2. Exit from the interaction

It is your right to walk away from any unpleasant or unhealthy interaction with an abusive person. Remember that you don't need a narcissist's permission to walk away.

Make the exit and interaction quick because the longer you stay engaged in the conversation, the longer you are late for your recovery, so to speak. The tricky part is that most times you don't want to just walk away from narcissists.

That would show them that you are defying or challenging their position. That would further infuriate them or mark you as someone with whom they need to get even. You don't want further aggravation than what you have already suffered.

There are subtle ways to exit a toxic conversation. Here are a couple of suggestions:

- Look at your watch or any time piece that is available and say, *"Oh my god, I'm late, got to go"* and then leave. Late for what? There is no need to explain anything.

- Pretend that you just got a call and start talking. It doesn't matter if there was really a call or not. Then tell your mother you have to go and just leave. The call is your excuse to stop talking to her and turn your attention to something else.

There are other things that you can do to exit from encounters with a narcissistic mother.

You can even make them up as you go. Think of it as your way of playing mind games on them since they have been playing mind games with you all along.

3. Talk like a politician

Do you notice how politicians talk on TV? They would be asked one thing but then they don't really answer the question directly. They just talk about the thing that they planned to discuss.

You can do the same thing when talking to a narcissist. It's like dodging the bullet and presenting your agenda at the same time. There are two things that you can do to get that effect.

First, whenever you are asked about something (usually something that your narcissist mother has a track record of belittling you or insulting you), just say "good" and then immediately talk about something else. When they do that again on another topic, say, "very well, actually" and then in the same sentence talk about another thing.

Next, here's something that you can do to shift the burden of proof from you to your mother. Do the same tactic as above but this time when you shift the topic under discussion, talk about something that your mother would love to talk about.

You already know what your narcissist is going to do, right? She will just go on and on about the subject, cheerleading herself along the way. At that point, you can enjoy your cup of tea or whatever beverage you were having and just ignore her prattle. When she catches her breath or runs out of things to say, then say goodbye.

4. Never overshare personal matters

You know the experience; you know what it's like to talk to a narcissist. It will always feel like an interrogation. Here's a big tip—don't explain, justify, or even overshare anything of a personal nature to a narcissist.

She'll just find another tool that she can use against you. Whenever she throws a critique, you can deflect it by saying, "Well, thank you for your opinion. I'll keep that in mind."

5. Call out what they did

Whenever your narcissistic mother insults you, calls you names, gets angry, interrupts the discussion, or puts people down (or any mind game they usually do), call it out and tell it to her face.

For example, when she insults your son or she insults you, say, "That sounded like an insult, we don't want any of that."

Another example would be when your mother hijacks the conversation and begins to talk about herself. At that point, you can interrupt her and say, "I noticed that each time I talk about something good I have done, you interrupt the conversation and talk about yourself."

She will fire back, but you don't need to engage her. In fact, after making that statement, you don't have to say anything else and whatever riveting statements she says after you called out the truth is actually irrelevant. No matter how she defends her position, you have already exposed her, which is something that narcissists aren't comfortable with.

You can then remind her of the boundaries you have set and then impose the consequence.

Remember that you will have to set boundaries over and over again. You will also have to remind your narcissistic mom of the rules and boundaries that you have set repeatedly.

Adjust your expectations. It will take a while before your narcissistic mother learns the rules and abides by them.

Chapter 10: Healthy Relationships Post-Narcissism

In the previous chapter, I mentioned that one of the steps for grieving the figurative loss of your mother is to find strength in people. Unfortunately, having a narcissistic mother cannot only isolate a daughter from previous relationships—it can hinder her ability to open up and make new ones.

That doesn't mean that it'll be impossible for you to have healthy relationships. You'll just need to work hard at each relationship you enter. In the end, it'll be worth it as each relationship fills you with love and a sense of belonging.

Friendships

Friendships are a crucial part of the human society, especially the social development of children. However, the daughter of a narcissistic mother is often deprived of this part of her childhood. Any time with a friend must be closely monitored by the narcissistic mother and only with the friends that she deems worthy of hanging out with her daughter—criteria that seems harder and harder to fulfill as time goes by. Eventually, the daughter will have few or no friends at all, and she will rarely go over to someone else's house unless her mother is there. After all, she might start to notice that her mother's behavior isn't quite normal when compared to her friends' mothers. Or, worse, she might start to like her friends' mothers more than her own, and that's a crack in the narcissistic mother's self-image that she just can't allow.

What does that mean for you, the narcissist's daughter?

Sadly, this isolation results in more than just a lonely childhood. You don't have the experience in making and maintaining friendships, and you are not emotionally primed for it. Still, there are things you can do for improving your preexisting friendships and for making new ones despite your mother's influence.

The first step is to reach out to whatever friends you might already have and touch base with them. This might surprise them as they will probably not know the real reason why you stopped talking to them or hanging out with them so much. Still, they'll be happy to hear from you.

You might experience anxiety from reaching out to them, wondering if your mother would approve or if she would love you if you just stopped hanging out with these kinds of people. Take a moment to remind yourself that this is just the way she has programmed you. No matter what you do, there will always be something you can do better. Don't feel bad for reaching out to your friends and for wanting to spend more time with them. She doesn't control you anymore.

Be warned, they might ask you why you're suddenly around more often or why you haven't been around more before now. When it comes to previous friendships, honesty is the best policy. Tell them about how your mother treated you. This will feel awkward at first, maybe even silly. You might fall back on that feeling that you're blowing it out of proportion and start scaling it back unintentional. Don't. It isn't just that your mother was strict or that she didn't like the friends you made. She put you down, controlled you, and isolated you. Don't sugarcoat it as you explain to your friends why it's been hard for you to put time into your friendship with them. You don't have to tell them everything, but don't make it seem less severe than it was.

Now, there will be some people who won't believe you. That's fine. They don't have to, and if they don't, they don't have to say thing about it to you. If they don't believe you and they bother you about it, though, then you don't need them. Look for the friends who support you during this time, even if they don't exactly understand or relate to what you're going through. You'd be surprised at how many you'll find.

When it comes to finding new friends, just follow the number one rule of this book: be patient with yourself. You need a support system and a sense of belonging when you heal, but none of this will happen overnight. You will need time to build your ability to trust, and you will be guarding your heart for a while. Take it slow. Start with big groups where you won't be the center of attention, like ones mentioned earlier, and then see if you'll connect with someone.

You don't need to find your new best friend right away, nor do you need to invite anyone to your apartment immediately or tell them anything personal. If they aren't in a support group for abuse survivors, you don't even have to tell them what you've been through with your mother. Just give them—and yourself—a chance. The more time you spend with them, the more comfortable you will be around them. The more comfortable you get with them, the easier it will be for you to open up.

Romantic Relationships

Romantic relationships make people vulnerable on a level that friendships don't. As a result, they're much harder for many people to form and maintain. For people who have been traumatized, like narcissist survivors, they're even harder. The daughter of a narcissistic mother will find it hard to open her hearts up in a way that is required to have a healthy, intimate relationship with a romantic partner. The ways in which her mother has put her down and belittled her will have dealt her confidence such a blow that she might still find herself unworthy of platonic love, let alone romantic love.

How, then, can you carry on a healthy romantic relationship after escaping from your narcissistic mother?

The ideal solution would be to wait until you have worked on yourself and reached a point of recovery and self-love where you are secure and confident. The problem is that life doesn't often work out so cleanly. You can mostly heal, but there will always be something that could trigger your insecurities and self-doubt, no matter how long it's been or how much work you've invested in yourself. Conversely, you might just meet someone that you don't want to miss out on getting to know before you've worked things out. Maybe you didn't realize your mother was an abusive narcissist until after you were already in a committed relationship.

Whatever the reason, there might come a time when you will have a partner and the two of you will have to work through your problems together. If you've been with them a while already, this won't be as much of a problem. They are already invested in you and your relationship, and they will do whatever is needed to make sure that everything from this point on is happy and healthy for the both of you.

A new relationship, however, will take more work. In the beginning, you will probably be more closed off, as you would be in a new friendship at this stage. Many people are for the first couple of dates, but if you aren't warming up to him after that, he might start to wonder what's wrong. Unlike with a new friend, you will need to tell a potential romantic partner about your narcissistic mother before things get too serious. It wouldn't be fair to either of you if you fall for each without having an idea about these kinds of problems. You also don't want him to be turned off by your coldness without first getting a chance to explain it to him.

You don't need to tell him the whole story. All you need to say is that you have some problems in your past that have given you emotional and trust issues, so it will take you some time to open up to anyone. If he has a problem with that, it's best that you find out now. If he doesn't, you might have found a new ally in your fight to reclaim your life from your mother's influence.

Relationships with Other Women

After I freed myself from my mother's grasp, I had a very hard time forming bonds with other women. Even women I had trusted before I realized what my mother was doing—aunts, cousins, female neighbors and friends—I had doubts about. I was weary of any compliments, sure that there were some sort of ulterior motive behind them. I wondered if these women really cared about me and was always waiting for the shoe to drop, even more so than with my male friends and relatives.

Fortunately, none of them gave up on me. They were patient, and I was lucky enough to find a new female role model in my paternal grandmother. She helped me to realize that not every woman is going to try to tear me down or use me to make themselves feel better. She showed me what a real friendship with a woman can be like. Eventually, I started to open up to the other women in my life and started to forge new female relationships as well.

Along with romantic relationships, relationships with other women can be the hardest to maintain as a direct result of your narcissistic mother's abuse. Because your mother was the ultimate model for all women in your mind, you become suspicious of all women, including the mothers that you have seen in healthy relationships with their daughters. You might worry about becoming a victim once again.

However, they are also one of the most important to establish during this time. Women can support other women in ways that their male friends and relatives just can't. Even my brother, who had lived through my mother alongside me, didn't understand the severity of the abuse or the ways in which it had affected me quite like my paternal grandmother did. He had his own scars that he dealt with in his own ways, but my relationships with my female friends and family made me feel loved and accepted, filling some of the hole that my mother had ripped in my heart.

All you have to do is remember what I said earlier: personalize, don't generalize. Not all women hurt you, just this one woman. It will be a hard distinction to make at first, but after you find just one woman to serve as a model for you and to support you throughout your process, you'll find yourself opening up more and more and generalizing less and less.

Relationships with Your Children

I personally avoided having children for as long as I felt I could because of my own upbringing. I didn't want to treat either my daughter or my son like my mother treated me and my brother, and I was almost willing to miss out on having children in order to prevent someone else from going through that. I was fortunate that my partner was very understanding and patient. Now we have a beautiful daughter and a handsome son, and both are being raised happy and healthy.

Believe it or not, this is actually a very common fear among the daughters of narcissistic mothers. They've heard that these sorts of things repeat, and so they assume that they will become just like their mothers if they ever become mothers.

Many of the women I have talked to have said that one of the things they worry about most when it comes to the long-term effects of their relationships with their mothers is that they will treat their daughters the same way their mothers treated them. Still, none of them were certain how to prevent this from occurring. It was as though they were second-guessing their ability to control such an outcome.

Fortunately, there are a few very easy ways to prevent this from happening while still being able to start a family of your own, if you want one.

- Get checked out by a psychiatrist

  Near the beginning of the book, I talked about how a narcissist can be diagnosed and treated by a psychiatrist or other mental health care professional. If you are truly concerned that you might treat your children the same way your mother treated you, talk with your therapist about it. Ask them to see if you might be a narcissist like your mother or if there's a possibility that you will project the pain from your upbringing onto your children.

If you don't currently see some sort of mental health care professional, consider seeing one as a proactive measure. It will also help you to heal from the wounds of your own abuse, which will hopefully make you less likely to project that pain onto your own children later on.

- Balance is key

One of the simplest answers is to pay attention to what you say to your children, particularly your daughter, and stop yourself if you find yourself insulting, belittling, or otherwise putting them down. Those insults are some of the most damaging parts of narcissistic abuse, and avoiding them will prevent you from repeating much of the damage that your mother inflicted on you.

However, that does not mean you should keep all negativity from your child at all times. There are times when a child needs to be exposed to certain kinds of negativity in order to grow as people.

One story from the women I spoke to stuck out to me as it illustrates both the abuse continuing and the results of the overcompensation that comes with it.

Let's take a look at Lupita's story:

"I put off having a family for a long time because of what I went through with my mother. I thought that if she was that way, odds were that I would be, too. My husband assured me that I'm not that kind of person, but I didn't believe him. Eventually he convinced me to try, and soon we had our little baby girl. As she got older, I was so worried about subconsciously treating her like my mother treated me that I did the exact opposite: I almost never said anything negative to her. I never even punished her. My husband had to handle all the punishments for the first seven years of her life, and thank goodness he did, or else who knows how spoiled she would've turned out.

There was a point when my husband pulled me aside and told me that I needed to start disciplining our daughter. He had told me this a million times before, but this time he said that if I didn't, he was worried that she would start to think that more than just eating dessert before dinner was OK. He told me that she had gotten in trouble at school for stealing the last pudding cup from another kid's tray and then throwing a tantrum when she was punished for it. He assured me that punishing her when she did something wrong would not make me the same as my mother. I knew then that he was right, and since then I have properly disciplined our daughter. She is a perfectly well-mannered young lady, and I'm proud to say that she'll never know the put-downs and abuse that I had to suffer through at her age."

Despite reassurances from her husband and no real reason to believe she would do this, Lupita worried that she would treat her daughter just like her mother treated her. In an effort to not tear down her daughter's confidence or make her daughter feel unloved, she avoided all negative language whatsoever, to the point that she wasn't even disciplining her child. Her daughter started going down a different bad route as a result, but fortunately Lupita's husband was able to catch it and get them all back on track before everything went awry.

Children need to be disciplined in order to learn what's right and what's wrong and grow as people. They also need to learn to recognize when someone is angry or otherwise upset, so it's unwise to shelter them from all forms of negativity altogether. What you need to do is treat your child well while also not putting them up on a pedestal. You don't want them to suffer like you did, but it's still your responsibility to make sure that they turn out to be responsible, moral adults.

- Treat your sons and daughters equally

While my mother abused both my brother and me, that is not always the case when it comes to families with narcissistic mothers. As I explained earlier, they might treat their sons well while abusing and putting down their daughters. That's why it's important to treat your sons and daughters equally, and I don't mean like how my mother treated my brother and me almost equally. Be consistent in how you punish and praise them and try not to play favorites.

You might not feel ready for all of these kinds of relationships right out of the gate, and that's okay. For now, focus on surrounding yourself with a support system of friends and family members that you already know and trust then expand your circle from there. It won't be easy opening up to people after what you've been through, but you'll get there.

Chapter 11: Mindfulness as a Healing Tool

Mindfulness meditation had been mentioned briefly in Chapter 5. In this chapter, we will cover in detail as to how this kind of meditation can help a daughter recover from the abuses of a narcissistic mother.

Back in 2014, researchers from the University of California, Davis, published a study of the effects of mindfulness meditation and practice. It was published in a journal which they aptly called *Mindfulness* [3]. The study involved participants of a three-day retreat. All subjects experienced abuse when they were little children—including narcissistic abuse.

The question they wanted to answer is whether mindfulness exercises, practices, and meditation can help these adults recover from abuse that have lasted for years. They were taught both loving kindness meditation as well as mindfulness meditation.

The study reported that after the three-day retreat, the participants experienced reduced emotional rumination and suppression. They achieved better emotional regulation and clarity. The women in particular have at least begun to approach their childhood experience with more self-awareness and less judgment.

What is Mindfulness?

Mindfulness is a practice or habit of maintaining an awareness of the things that are currently happening to you. It is like being zoned into the now. With careful practice and improved mental, emotional, and spatial awareness (which you gain from mindfulness exercises), you gain a moment-by-moment awareness of things.

You become more aware of your surrounding environment, your bodily sensations, your feelings, your memories, and your thoughts. With that as a practice, you take on a neutral stance—a non-judgmental observer and thus taking everything with a rather nurturing point of view.

Mindfulness isn't something new. It has its roots in Zen Buddhism, and it has been said that Buddha practiced it in order to be aware of his own experience and there continued until he reached a state called nirvana.

Nowadays, mindfulness is not just religious or mystical mumbo jumbo. It is actually a therapeutic practice used by thousands. While you might not reach the mystical state of nirvana, you'll at least get something close to it: a state of peace and clarity of mind.

The secular side of mindfulness meditation started in 1979 with the work of Jon Kabat-Zinn at the University of Massachusetts Medical School. His program has been adopted today in veteran centers, hospitals, prisons, schools, and others. It has the potential to help people with anxiety and other similar issues.

Putting Mindfulness to Practice

The wonderful thing about mindfulness is that you don't need to sit down like Buddha or some ancient monk surrounded by nature in order to do it. You don't even need to close your eyes to practice it. You can take a walk in the park or walk your way to the office and do mindfulness exercises along the way.

Jon Kabat-Zinn once described it as *"living your life as if it really mattered, moment by moment by moment by moment."*

Today, it's more than just a kind of meditation; it's a lifestyle and a day-to-day practice.

Key Components of Mindfulness as a Daily Practice

- Pay attention to the way you breathe, especially when you are under stress or when you feel really intense emotions.

- Pay attention to and tune into your sensations. Where is the wind blowing on you? Where is the water from the shower hitting? How does the chair feel while you're sitting at work? What are the actual sounds you're hearing from the music being played? What does the food taste like with each bite you take? Awareness of your sensations is a key to this practice.

- Recognize that feelings, emotions, and memories are only fleeting. They are like storms. They come and eventually they will go. You don't have to react to them because they come and go whether you react or not.

- Pay attention to your senses. What do you smell in the restaurant? How does the fabric of your shirt feel? How does that look from your boss make you feel? It's not really that threatening, is it?

Mindfulness Exercises You Can Try Now

Here are two mindfulness exercises that you can try right now. After trying them, I recommend that you find a therapist or a mindfulness coach to give you some guidance along the way as you grow and heal.

Mindful Breathing – Breathing is a pretty common element in any form of meditation. The good news is that you can do it anywhere. You could be sitting in your cubicle at work and practice this breathing technique for just a minute or two. Here are the steps:

1. Sit on a chair and get as comfy as you can.

2. Rest your hands where they can be comfortable.

3. Relax and allow yourself to notice every part of your body.

4. Take a mental note of every sensation as you sit comfortably on your chair.

5. Pay attention to your breathing.

6. Answer this question in your mind—where is the air entering your body?

7. Are you breathing from your abdomen or are you breathing from your chest?

8. Notice how the air feels as it passes through your nostrils, chest, and as it enters and exits your lungs.

9. As you pay attention to your breathing, notice that your mind will wander from time

to time. Forgive yourself when that happens.

10. Gently redirect your attention back to your breathing again.

11. Take more relaxing breaths and observe them.

12. You will also notice that painful memories of your childhood might creep into your thoughts. A few things may trigger them, like the music being played, an image you may be seeing now, or maybe it just comes up like it has a mind of its own.

13. Again, observe the memory. Observe the emotion. Don't judge the memory, don't judge the emotion. Just observe.

14. See that it comes and then the memory just fades away.

15. Now, forgive yourself and gently bring your focus back to your breathing.

16. After about a minute or two, you can decide if you want to continue doing this for a few minutes more.

17. Remember that it's all up to you. You have the power to choose.

Body Scan – This mental exercise is kind of similar to the one above. The big difference is that you move your focus from your breathing to something bigger—your body. Other mindfulness exercises are like that, you train your mental focus on the world around you, but you should do that only when you're ready. Start with the small things like your breathing and, this time, your body.

Here's how you do it:

1. You can do this exercise whether you're sitting, standing, or even while walking.

2. Do it only when you're comfortable—in case you're walking, do it in a non-stressful place like a park or something.

3. Take a few slow and deep breaths.

4. Pay attention to the relaxing feeling as you breathe slowly and deeply.

5. Pay attention to your feet.

6. How do they feel? If you are walking, take a mental note of how they feel when they fall on the ground.

7. If you are sitting, pay attention to how your back feels against the back rest. Make adjustments to make you feel comfortable.

8. If you're standing up or walking, pay attention to if your back is hunched or if you are standing straight.

9. Adjust your posture to make things more comfortable.

10. Pay attention to your hands—are they tense or not?

11. Pay attention to your knees, hips, and other parts of your body.

12. As you observe the sensations you feel in the different parts of your body, notice that

your mind will wander or some distant memory might also come along to disrupt your mental work.

13. Treat them the same way you treated the rest of your body. You observe them. Watch them come and go.

14. Forgive yourself for straying.

15. Gently move your attention back to the body scan.

16. You can go about it from head to toe or from your foot going up to your head. It's all up to you.

17. Notice how relaxing it feels.

18. After 15 minutes of this, you can stop or continue for another 15 minutes. It's all up to you. You're free.

Given the keys and the practices mentioned above, you can use mindfulness exercises whenever you find the chance to do them. You could be sitting in a bus on the way home and practice mindfulness. As you do it from day to day, eventually you will get an appreciation for the things you have now.

After you have tried it several times, I recommend that you find a therapist that includes mindfulness in therapy sessions. That way, you can learn more exercises and put them to practice in your day-to-day life.

The road to recovery is long, but with perseverance, patience, and forgiveness of self, you can find healing and appreciate the wonderful opportunity at life that is totally yours now that you are free.

Recovery and Healing Toolbox

In this section, I would like to share some of the tools that helped me along the way in my road to recovery and healing. Much of the activities, ideas, and exercises included here are drawn from the things that therapists suggested I do.

I have done a lot of other exercises, not just the ones mentioned here. However, I only included these things below because they were the ones that worked best for me. I'm not guaranteeing that they will work for you, too.

That is why I recommend that you work with your therapist. Talk to them about the activities and tools below and see if they will approve of them, too. Give them a try. If they work, then it's one step forward in your own journey as well.

Tool #1—Affirmations

I have covered affirmations in passing in this book, so I would like to go over them in more detail here.

Believe it or not, I felt silly at first when affirmations for narcissistic abuse victims were introduced to me. I thought that they were just words. However, I learned that there is power in words.

Remember how your narcissistic mother manipulated you? She used words. Words are that powerful. I remember my mom emphasized three important points and used very powerful words to ingrain them in my mind.

She made me remember that:

1. Love is earned.

2. The real me didn't matter—what other people thought of me mattered.

3. My purpose is to make people look up to Mom.

I was reminded of this line from the movie *V for Vendetta*:

"...words will always retain their power. Words offer the means to meaning, and for those who will listen, the enunciation of truth."

Words are powerful. And in my experience, affirmations are powerful because they enunciate the truth. I was made to believe lies about myself throughout my childhood, and it took positive affirmative words to rebuild me from within.

I suggest that you find 5 to 10 minutes in the morning before you do anything else. Don't go to the kitchen to make breakfast. Don't go to the shower and don't start preparing for work.

I provided a short set of affirmations earlier, and here I would like to give you a few more. I suggest that the first thing you should do in the morning is to go to the mirror, look yourself in the eye, and say the following truths to yourself:

Affirmations Set 1

- I am healing, one day at a time, one step at a time.

- The past is behind me, I focus on the now and the future.

Affirmations Set 2

- I am loved.

- I'm a lovable person.

- I deserve affection.

- I deserve care.

- I deserve respect.

Affirmations Set 3

- I prioritize self-care.

- I trust my own mind.

- I have set firm boundaries.

- I stick to these boundaries.

Affirmations Set 4

- I have my family.

- I have my friends.

- They support me.

- I am not alone.

Affirmations Set 5

NOTE: this one I used when I got an email, text, or any other sort of communication from my narcissistic mother.

- I have set my boundaries.

- I don't have to be afraid.

- I don't need to reply.

- My silence is my protection.

- I have the right to be free from abuse.

These affirmations will help you adjust your internal monologue. The affirmations I have provided above will help take your mind away from a state of helplessness and will move your mind into a position of empowerment.

You can always edit the lines of these affirmations. In fact, you can even just take one line from each of these sets and repeat them over and over like a kind of mantra. Just make sure that the line picked is very meaningful to you.

Tool #2—Adult Coloring Books

You can buy these coloring books from a lot of sources. I bought mine from Amazon. Are they helpful? Well, consider the following:

"...making and creating artwork is used to explore feelings, reconcile emotional conflicts, foster self-awareness, manage behavior and addictions, develop social skills, improve reality orientation, reduce anxiety and increase self-esteem."

That's from the American Art Therapy Association. I have found that these coloring books help with anxiety relief, they're inexpensive, and they help release repressed emotions. These coloring books are also less intimidating, that is, if you're like me and haven't tried any form of art in your entire life.

Tool #3—Music Therapy

Music therapy will first begin with the help of a therapist. I was informed of this methodology and I can personally vouch for it. Again, I am no musical virtuoso and so at first my therapist did all the music playing for me.

I eventually joined in via singing along and other stuff. Then my therapist suggested drumming. I couldn't believe how fun it was. It helped ease away the feelings of isolation and alienation. It helped me release emotional trauma. It also induced relaxation. If you want to read more about drumming and music therapy's effects, click here. [https://www.ncbi.nlm.nih.gov/pmc/articles/PMC1447805]

If you're interested in trying this out, I suggest that you sign up with a music therapy center, like Newport Academy (click here). [https://www.newportacademy.com]

Tool #4—Goal Setting

Goal setting has helped me regain a clearer focus about what I want to do next with my life. Living with a narcissistic mother is more like living only for her. Now that that is no longer my purpose, I needed direction.

Goal setting also helped me fine tune my decision-making capabilities. It helped me realize that I can decide on something and achieve it. It helped me realize that I can achieve and do the things that my mom told me I couldn't do.

Here's how you do it.

1. Grab your journal/diary and make a life audit.

2. List all the things that you missed out on, things you were told you couldn't do, things that you were afraid to do.

3. You can even include all the fun things that you have always wanted to do.

4. Review your list – find one thing that you can do this weekend. It can be anything from playing golf, going to a bar, a spa, go swimming, karaoke night, scuba diving, or just going out with your friends. It can be anything.

5. Plan that thing this weekend. Grab a friend – it will help to have some company along.

6. Prepare everything three days before.

7. Go for it on the day you planned it, no matter what.

8. Keep going for it no matter how scary, discouraging, or even how silly it is making you feel.

9. The important thing is that you were there and you did it and it felt fun. Oh yeah, make sure to take pictures as a memento of the experience.

10. At the end of the day, make a review of the experience. Was it fun, entertaining, interesting, or was it something that you would like to do again?

11. Write everything down in your journal or post it on your blog.

12. Repeat everything from step 4.

Tool #5—The 3-3-3 Rule

This is a trick that was taught to me by my psychiatrist which became my go-to tool whenever I feel a panic attack or when anxiety sets in. Here's how it goes:

1. When you feel panicky or when you immediately feel anxious, look around you.

2. Name the first three things that you see.

3. Listen for things around you, name three things that you hear.

4. Finally, move three parts of your body. It can be any part—your hands, arms, forearms, fingers, toes, neck, flex your stomach muscles, anything.

5. Repeat from step 1.

This exercise is also a mindfulness exercise, actually. It helps center your mind on the present moment.

Tool #6—Comedy Night!

As the saying goes, "laughter is the best medicine." Well, the Anxiety and Depression Association of America (ADAA) confirms that humor is a clinically validated means for relieving stress.

It works because when you laugh and enjoy some comedy your body releases beta-endorphins and it also reduces your blood pressure. Your body also releases neuropeptides that help boost your immune system.

Again, bring a friend (or friends) along so you can laugh out loud with someone that you are comfortable with. If you're not too keen on watching stand-up comedy with a live audience, then you can just watch a comedy show on TV. Again, do it with friends or family. It will help make the experience more meaningful.

Tool #7—Aroma Therapy

I'm not sure if aroma therapy will work for everyone. It worked for me, so I suggest that you try it. Other than that, aroma therapy is backed by scientific studies. You're going to need either an aroma therapy inhaler or a diffuser.

The inhaler will cost you anything from $8 to $20. So, they're really cheap. There are sets that will cost you a thousand bucks but who needs those expensive brands anyway, right? An aroma therapy diffuser will cost you anywhere from $20 to $300.

Follow the instructions with regard to the ratio of the essential oils to the carrier oil. I carry my inhaler with me all the time and use it whenever I feel anxiety coming in.

These tools for recovery and healing have helped me a lot in my journey to recovery. I hope that they will benefit you, too.

One Last Reminder Before Conclusion

Have you grabbed your free resource?

A lot of information has been covered in this book. As previously shared, I've created a simple mind map that you can use *right away* to easily understand, quickly recall and readily use what you've learned in this book.

If you've not grabbed it...

Click Here To Get Your Free Resource

Alternatively, here's the link:

https://viebooks.club/freeresourcemind-mapfordidmynarcissisticmotherloveme

Your Free Resource Is Waiting..

Get Your Free Resource Now!

Conclusion

I'd like to thank you and congratulate you for transiting my lines from start to finish.

I hope this book was able to help you to find the tools you need to find peace, forgiveness, and healing from narcissistic abuse.

The next step is to find a therapist that has worked extensively with patients of childhood trauma. You should also continue practicing mindfulness, cool processing, setting healthy barriers, and all the tips and recommendations made in this book.

I wish you the best of luck!

Sincerely,

Nanette Abigail

P.S.

If you've found this book helpful in any way, a review on Amazon is greatly appreciated.

This means a lot to me, and I'll be extremely grateful.

Notes

[1] Millon, T. et al. "Personality disorders in modern life." *Wiley* (2004): 343

[2] Zuern, J.D.. "Freud: on narcissism." *CriticaLink, University of Hawaii* (1998)

[3] Caldwell, Jon G., & Shaver, Phillip R.. "Promoting attachment-related mindfulness and compassion: a wait-list-controlled study of women who were mistreated during childhood." *Mindfulness* (2014): 1-15

Related Books That Might Benefit You

Emotional Abuse Recovery: Men & Women Suffering in Silence – Emotionally Abusive, Destructive Relationship or Marriage with Manipulative, Toxic People (Healthy Healing and Recovering from Trauma)

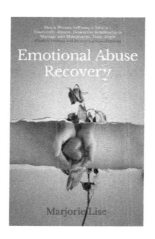

<u>Stop Suffering In Silence & Finally Heal From Emotionally Abusive Relationship With The Help Of This POWERFUL Guide!</u>

Are you constantly feeling emotionally tortured and betrayed by someone you used to love and adore?

Do you see no point in even trying to get out because your abusive partner has taken full control of your life?

Do you feel suffocated and helpless because it just seems like no one understands, or knows how to help you?

If you want to stop all these in your life, then keep reading...

Going through, and subsequently healing from emotional abuse is easier said than done. Most times, abuse victims feel blamed for staying or getting themselves into that kind of relationship in the first place.

Abuse survivor turned domestic violence advocate, Marjorie Lise, knows this story all too well. Lise had stayed with her abusive partner for an entire decade, before realizing that she deserved better. In her book, she talks about how she was able to successfully stop suffering in silence and finally escape her abuser, with the hope that her experience will inspire others to take back control of their lives, too.

Lise wants people like you to know that there is HOPE!

Emotional Abuse Recovery, the only book you'll ever need to get out of an emotionally abusive relationship and finally start to heal!

Here's a taste of what you'll discover inside *Emotional Abuse Recovery*:

- *Unmistakable signs to watch out for* to accurately recognize and effectively address toxic relationships, manipulative people and emotional abusers

- *Destructive ways that emotional manipulation* can affect a person for the rest of their life

- *Detailed and clear guidelines in taking the first steps* in dealing with your abuser, starting the healing process, and taking back control of your life

- *Proven methods in creating an air-tight safety plan* that will help you get out of EVERY sticky, abusive situation

- *Effective techniques to maximize the positive effects* that guided journaling can do in easing negative emotions stemming from abuse

- *Actionable tips that help you be and stay strong during the critical recovery stage*, so you won't feel the need to give in or go back to your abuser ever again

- *Highly reliable, helpful, and easily accessible resources* that you can use whenever you need emotional, physical, and mental help

And much, much more...

If you're ready to finally heal from your trauma, experience emotionally healthy relationships that you deserve, and say goodbye to your abusive torturer for good, now is the time.

Co-Dependency: The Crazy Codependent in Toxic Relationship - The Codependency Cure, Healing & Recovery from Trauma for Emotionally Healthy Love Relationships with Partner, Parent, Mother or Father

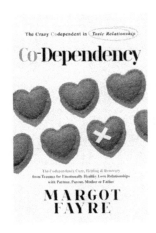

<u>This POWERFUL Guide Will Help You Overcome & Recover From Codependent Relationship & Cultivate Your Own Growth!</u>

Do you often feel guilty when you're not able to help someone who completely depends on you?

Are you feeling like you don't have the freedom to explore opportunities for growth?

Do you feel like you can't live up to your full potential because you have to take care of everyone's needs before your own?

If you want to stop all these in your life, then keep reading...

A codependent relationship can feel like a burden on the person bearing the brunt of other people's problems. Being in it often leave you feeling used, unappreciated and angry. Most times, you feel almost forced to help certain people solve their problems as you feel compelled to pacify their negative emotions, give various suggestions, or offer unwanted advice.

Margot Fayre, Doctor of Psychology, knows this all too well. Once in a codependent relationship herself, she knows how frustrating and limiting all of this can feel like. This was the impetus that drove her to write her book, so she can help people like you overcome codependency using science-backed insights.

Are you ready to find out if you're being taken advantage of, end your codependent relationship, and finally set yourself free?

Co-Dependency, the only book you'll ever need to finally overcome and recover from a codependent partner, friend or relative who hampers your growth, and start cultivating emotionally healthy relationships.

Here's a taste of what you'll discover inside *Co-Dependency*:

- *Definitely understand what it means to be in a codependent relationship* so you can make the necessary life changes using SIMPLE techniques

- *Quickly discover what your triggers are* so you know how your mind works and EASILY put an end to your codependence issues

- *Firmly set your personal boundaries* and COURAGEOUSLY assert yourself so you no longer need to depend on anybody

- **Effectively make changes within** using mindfulness and practical methods based on PROVEN psychology principles

- **Take absolute, full responsibility for your own emotions** and resolve conflicts using FIELD-TESTED methods

- **Fast-track your journey in recovering from co-dependency** by figuring out and tapping into your GREATEST strengths

- **Become a better partner, friend and family member** by becoming a GREAT team player and advocate

And much, much more...

If you're ready to finally take back control of your life, live up to your maximum potential, and say goodbye to your controlling relationships, now is the time.

Narcissistic Abuse Recovery in Toxic Relationship: Healing Love & Recovering from Covert Narcissism, Manipulation & Trauma - Dealing with Abusive Narcissist Partner, Family, Parent, Mother or Father

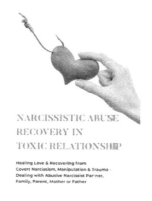

NARCISSISTIC ABUSE
RECOVERY IN
TOXIC RELATIONSHIP

Healing Love & Recovering from
Covert Narcissism, Manipulation & Trauma -
Dealing with Abusive Narcissist Partner,
Family, Parent, Mother or Father

NAILA FARRAH

<u>This LIFE-CHANGING Guide Will Teach You How To Cut Narcissist Out Of Your Life So They Can Never Hurt You Again!</u>

Do you often feel like you're condoning abusive behavior from people who claim to love you?

Have you stopped doing the things you love be-cause someone in your life criticizes you for do-ing them?

Do you feel suffocated and overwhelmed because you are under constant undeserved scrutiny?

If you want to stop all these in your life, then keep reading...

Dealing with narcissists can be emotion-ally and psychologically exhausting and traumatic. Most narcissists feel entitled to eve-ryone's attention, as well as exploit others with-out guilt or shame. Often times, the victims never really know what hit them until it's too late.

Award-winning author, Naila Farrah, knows a thing or two about falling victim to a nar-cissist. In fact, her experience was even more heartbreaking since the abuser was her own fa-ther — someone who is supposed to make her feel safe and loved. Once she had stopped condoning his bad behavior, her world changed for the better and this paved the way to her narcissistic abuse recovery. All of a sudden, it was like a heavy weight had been taken off her shoulders. She became happier, brighter, and content... and she wishes the same things for you, too!

In her book, Farrah aims to empower people like you to take back control and start living life free from toxic, controlling people.

***Narcissistic Abuse Recovery in Toxic Relationship*, the only book you'll ever need to discover the reality of covert narcissism and learn how to spot a narcissist with narcissistic personality disorder before they start hurting you!**

Here's a taste of what you'll discover inside *Narcissistic Abuse Recovery in Toxic Relationship*:

- ***Swiftly learn the signs to watch out for*** so you can SKILLFULLY stop a narcissist from coming into your life and creating chaos

- ***Easily find out if you're in a relationship with a narcissist*** so you can EFFECTIVELY deal with them and kick start your own narcissistic abuse recovery

- ***Effectively cut toxic people out of your life*** using this one FOOLPROOF method that will change the course of your life

- ***Fast-track your healing from a narcissistic relationship*** and get your life back in a snap using PROVEN techniques and tools

- ***Discover the exact ways*** you can QUICKLY heal your brain from all the emotional turmoil and trauma and reverse whatever damage has been done

- ***Use SCIENCE-BACKED, practical advice*** so you can FINALLY move forward and start a new life away from your narcissistic abuser

- ***Immediately free yourself*** from a narcissistic person's grip and start cultivating healthier relationships with a few SIMPLE steps

And much, much more...

If you're ready to finally learn how to deal with a narcissist, break free from the emotional and psychological chaos, start your narcissistic abuse recovery, and live a happier, contented and fulfilled life, now is the time.